T0313853

Emerging Socialities and Subjectivities in
Twenty-First-Century Healthcare

Emerging Socialities and Subjectivities in Twenty-First-Century Healthcare

Edited by Bernhard Hadolt and Anita Hardon

Amsterdam University Press

Cover image: https://unsplash.com/photos/6-jTZysYY_U?photo_info_popover=is_visible

Cover design: Coördesign, Leiden
Lay-out: Crius Group, Hulshout
Printed and bound by CPI Group (UK) Ltd, Croydon, CR0 4YY

Amsterdam University Press English-language titles are distributed in the US and Canada by
the University of Chicago Press.

ISBN	978 94 6298 277 2
e-ISBN	978 90 4853 281 0 (pdf)
DOI	10.5117/9789462982772
NUR	882

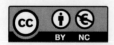

Table of Contents

Part III NEW SOCIALITIES AND SUBJECTIVITIES IN CARE

Part IV NEW SUBJECTIVITIES, SOCIALITIES, AND THE MEDIA

Emerging Socialities and Subjectivities in Twenty-First-Century Healthcare

Introduction

Anita Hardon and Bernhard Hadolt

Health care, conceived broadly as institutionalized as well as non-institutionalized forms of tending to sickness and health, is undergoing transformations at a high speed and with unprecedented outcomes. Accelerated global flows of medical goods and services, ongoing economization of health in the context of cutbacks of health-related public expenditures, demographic changes and the 'greying' of societies, as well as new and re-emergent pandemics affect the health care landscapes in the 21st century. In addition, new actors in health care policy making emerge, and we are confronted with a professionalization of 'traditional' healing services. Moreover, the ready availability of vast health information via the Internet, social networks, and other currents contributes to and is part of rapidly changing health care constellations. This edited volume brings together medical anthropologists who describe these transformations with a focus on the new socialities and subjectivities that emerge. Their contributions were presented at the seventh biannual conference of the Medical Anthropology At Home (MAAH) network, held in 2012 in Driebergen, the Netherlands, which was hosted by the Social Science and Global Health research priority of the University of Amsterdam and led by Bernhard Hadolt and Anita Hardon. The conference was held in honour of Els van Dongen, who launched MAAH with a conference in the Netherlands in 1998 and who passed away in 2009.

The relations between patients and healers have been an important focus in medical anthropology, providing insights into power dynamics and divergences in meaning and practice. Contemporary health socialities, however, no longer only involve doctors/healers and patients, but also scientists, health goods suppliers, NGOs, policy-makers, media, and others. The ways in which people nowadays relate to each other in health care have been framed as biosociality, and as biological, genetic, and therapeutic citizenship. Health-related socialities are intimately connected to how individuals position and experience themselves in relation to each other, to their bodies, to medical technologies, to health and disease, and to health care. How do changing health care constellations and emerging socialities affect patient subjectivities and moralities? Which new subject positions become available, and how? In what ways can we examine and explore these changing subjectivities? Which social science theories and concepts provide useful points of departure? What new theoretical understandings emerge from current work in these fields? The contributions to this book provide empirical case studies that reflect on these questions, while outlining the transformations in health policy that are emerging and more specifically the role of the Internet in contemporary health care.

Revisiting concepts

The first section of this edited volume revisits theoretical concepts that have shaped 21st-century thinking about the ways people relate to each other in health care. In the first section, Roberta Raffaetà challenges the popularity of the concept of biosociality, arguing that it is a valuable but only partial representation of the relationship between the domains of biology and culture. She presents the case of parental groups that are critical of certain aspects of paediatric vaccinations in Italy, demonstrating how these groups affirm the priority of what they conceive as nature over culture. In the second chapter of this section, Franz Graf examines a new sociality being created by Europeans attracted to *curanderismo* (the practice of Latin American folk medicine), which he discusses in relation to scholarship on the 'new animism'. Pursuing a more meaningful relationship with the whole natural world, these students and recipients of indigenous healing seek to combat the alienation of the neoliberal, individualized body.

New policies and programs

The second section of the book focuses on new health policies and programs and how they affect and are shaped by health socialities and subjectivities in diverse and sometimes unexpected ways. Bernhard Hadolt and Monika Gritsch present a comparative analysis of the societal acceptance of human papillomavirus (HPV) vaccination marketing. They describe how HPV vaccination initially was overwhelmingly embraced in Japan and only tepidly received in Austria, arguing that policy making and public debates intersect with global drug marketing strategies. They further argue that HPV vaccination marketing strategies are not only tailored to local circumstances but also the reverse is the case, sometimes with rapid shifts in unexpected ways. Prachatip Kata's contribution focuses on how new government policies in Thailand shape health subjectivities. He describes how people with physical disabilities in Thailand are constructed as 'ambiguous citizens' by a combination of government policy and Theraveda Buddhist precepts. He argues that in this Thai biopolitics of impairment, 'good citizens' are those who contribute to the economic health of the nation state; those who cannot, because of their karma, must depend on the compassion of others. Bodil Ludvigsen describes how in Denmark, in stark contrast to the economic context of Thailand, social relations between nurses and elderly home-care recipients change as a result of a turn toward market-based health care. Computer programs now organize nurses' daily schedules, making it much less common for nurses to see the same patient over time. Good nurses are those who manage to do their work in an efficient way. And finally, Ivo Quaranta describes a new kind of migrant care in Italy. He examines how 'agency can take place from within biopower', as illustrated in the case of a new, anthropologically informed Socio-Cultural Consultation Centre in Bologna. Patients co-construct the meaning of their health situation in consultations with a variety of health professionals, moving beyond illness narration to empowerment.

New socialities and subjectivities in care

The four contributions in the third section of the book further reflect on how new subjectivities and socialities emerge in encounters between carers and recipients of care in diverse institutional settings. Stemming from multi-sited research on Muslim migrants in perinatal care in Montreal, Sylvie Fortin and Josiane Le Gall discuss socialities in the context of migration, with special attention to the changing role of fathers, and how these socialities are involved in the clinical encounter. They point out that gender relationships and inequalities shape clinical discourses and practices, despite (or due to) a greater involvement of the father in the perinatal sphere. Julia Thiesbonenkamp-Maag describes pastoral care in Germany, showing how hospital chaplains' ways of relating to patients, their relatives, and medical staff are based on an ethics of care in which the chaplains try, through the act of 'witnessing', to see the whole picture rather than just repairing people. Examining the care related to terminal illnesses, and amyotrophic lateral sclerosis (ALS) in particular, Martine Verwey in her contribution takes a longitudinal approach to describing health-related subjectivities. She discusses how, as the disease progresses, tensions can emerge about what constitutes 'good care'. Using the case of her late husband, she demonstrates how medical professionals try to balance care for the ill person with care for the caregiver, but in doing so can begin to treat patients more like objects than self-determining subjects. Finally Claudie Haxaire focuses on doctors' perception of the patient and the patient's social context in western Brittany, France. She shows how social context is the key factor in determining whether or not a doctor defines a patient's psychotropic drug use as evidence of addiction.

New media

The two contributions to the fourth and last section of this book focus on the role of the Internet in the formation of health subjectivities and socialities. Taking up the French debate on the merits of self-medication, Sylvie Fainzang delineates two 'cybernetic socialities': those who seek or share information about medications, and those who argue for and against self-medication. She proposes the notion of 'health sociality' to describe these web-based exchanges, all of which share a concern with the social, physiological, and legal possibilities of managing one's own body. Finally, Lina Masana examines how the Internet, with its web forums, chat rooms, and other forms of social media, offers the possibility of new forms of sociality for people who are chronically ill and homebound in Catalonia, Spain. She shows how people use the Internet as a means to transcend the physical barriers imposed on them by their illness in order to actively engage in a virtual social life of mutual care and thus overcome isolation and mutual care.

The goal of collecting these case studies is to explore recent organizational and technological changes in health care and how the subjectivities and socialities of both patients and health care workers are impacted. Situated in diverse locales, these twelve stories provide the reader with a glimpse into new dynamics, as patients' groups shape policy, states affect pharmaceutical markets, software defines nurse-patient relationships, and the Internet connects isolated patients. Together, the cases make the resilient argument that not only are new socialities emerging, but new ethics and moralities are being forged and contested alongside them.

Part I
REFLECTING THEORY—Revisiting concepts

1   Biosociality extended

The case of parental groups campaigning against paediatric vaccinations in Italy

Roberta Raffaetà

Various studies in medical anthropology (for example, Lock and Nguyen, 2010) have illustrated that biomedical diagnoses do not pertain to the realm of nature but to culture and politics, arguing that biomedical knowledge is a flexible tool that may be used to support or refute specific world views and practices. In particular, biomedical technologies have been considered as a particular way of crafting nature. As Strathern (1992) has famously argued, since nature has been assisted by technology, it can no longer constitute a prior ontological status to culture. Similarly, others (Haraway, 1997; Rose, 2001) have showed how culture and nature are increasingly densely intertwined and how difficult is to distinguish the natural from the artificial. Within this landscape, Rabinow (1992) has proposed the concept of biosociality to refer to the collective identities emerging from biomedical categories. In the concept of biosociality, culture has primacy over nature as it provides the model for nature in a biotechnological age.

In this chapter, I challenge this valuable but partial representation of the relationship between the domains of biology and culture by illustrating the case of parental groups who are critical of certain aspects of paediatric vaccinations in Italy. After describing these groups as specific forms of sociality (a social grouping that provides certain subject positions, beyond the categorization of certain people) (Whyte, 2009), I illustrate how these parental groups affirm the priority of nature over culture, thus extending the notion of biosociality. The prefix 'bio' in the term 'biosociality' refers to a dimension of life—its indeterminacy and potentiality—that is usually disqualified by theoretical approaches that conflate nature and culture. To unravel the theoretical and political consequences posed by the case of parental groups, I draw on Monica Greco's reading of George Canguilhem's distinction between normativity and normality, and on Giorgio Agamben's analysis of the relationship between *zoē* and *bios*.

The study

My interest in the topic of paediatric vaccinations began with the birth of my daughter in 2008 and the invitation, received a few weeks after the birth, to take her for vaccination at the local public health centre. Having done research on immunology and the immune system in previous years, I had some doubts about vaccination and I started to search the Internet for information. I also contacted a local parental group, which provided me with information and support in deciding whether or not to have my daughter vaccinated. The more I learned about vaccination and parental groups, the more I became interested in the topic, transforming my personal wandering in search of information into a more systematic inquiry.

The methodology employed for this study was qualitative and ethno-graphic. Initially, I reviewed the main Italian online resources provided by parents' organizations critical of certain aspects of vaccination policy. After establishing contact with the representatives of a local organization, I attended their meetings for about two years. On one of these occasions, I publicly explained my research objectives and asked for volunteers to be interviewed. I explained that I was looking for people (including doctors) willing to tell me their ideas and/or experiences concerning paediatric vaccination (independent of their decision whether or not to vaccinate). I interviewed 4 doctors and 21 families, 5 of which I followed in their consultations with medical professionals at the Department of Preventive Medi-cine—Hygiene and Public Health of the local health authority (Azienda Sanitaria Locale). Parental groups suggested that parents pursue medical consultations as an opportunity to voice their scepticism towards vaccines. In addition, I also conducted informal interviews with Italian friends, most of whom had vaccinated their children. Informed consent was obtained for the interviews, recordings, and my observations at consultations. Interviews were transcribed verbatim and field notes were analysed thematically.

The sociality of parental groups

In Italy there are four compulsory vaccinations, against tetanus, hepatitis B, diphtheria, and poliomyelitis, and vaccination is also recommended against meningitis, pertussis, and measles. If the compulsory and recom-mended vaccinations are added together, Italian babies receive up to 27 vaccines (including boosters) within the first three years of their lives (Serravalle, 2009, p. 9). These are administered as a hexavalent vaccine, meaning a single injection of six combined vaccines (four compulsory and two recommended).

Since 2000, Italian legislation has defined vaccination as compulsory but not to be enforced. However, in practice, most Italian families hardly have an option in the matter: they are subject to what can be termed the moral 'imperative to vaccinate' and most parents do not even consider the possibility of refusing. In Italy, the vaccination of children is considered a normal, routine act of good and responsible parenting, in the same way that breathing is the normal behaviour of an organism; and just as living beings breathe even if they do not decide to do so, most parents in Italy do not choose to vaccinate their children, they simply do it. The packaging of six vaccines in one injection partly conceals the fact that two of them are not mandatory. Parents do not choose to have their children vaccinated, nor do they choose which vaccines to have injected: everything is already decided for them. Vaccination is catalysed by the laying out of a particular seemingly self-evident procedure: without any action on the part of the parents, each baby is assigned a schedule for vaccinations, and parents are reminded about dates by letter. This is because vaccinations are national public health initiatives, and, as such, they are promoted as both safe and effective. The common rhetoric, inspired by the achievements of immunology in the early days (Martin and Marshall, 2003; Moulin, 1991), describes vaccines as 'one of the greatest public health success stories' (Poland and Jacobson, 2001, p. 2440).

Parents considering forgoing vaccination have usually had experience with adverse reactions to vaccines or have heard about such reactions from friends or media reports. The reasons put forward by parents' groups to justify non-vaccination or to alter the standard vaccine schedule (vaccinating at a later age, or administering single selected vaccines), are many and interrelated. However, they mainly have to do with concerns about safety and effectiveness (Benatti, Ambrosi, and Rosa, 2006; Gava, 2008; Raffaetà, 2012, p. 13; Serravalle, 2009). The first parental group concerned with vaccination to appear in Italy was the Lega per la Libertà delle Vaccinazioni (League for Freedom Regarding Vaccination), which was founded in 1985 in Brescia (a city near Milan) by a group of parents and doctors in response to the forced vaccination of the Tremante family. In 1981 the parents asked that their twins be exempted from vaccination, as their first child died after being vaccinated. They were refused exemption; following vaccination, one of the Tremante twins died and the other became paraplegic. Since 1993, the Lega per la Libertà delle Vaccinazioni has been seen as a model for other parental groups, including Vaccinareinformati (Association for Informed

Vaccination), a group I followed and participated in as part of my research, located in the province of Trento.

Parents join parental groups not in response to a diagnosis—whether of a genetic variation (Rabinow, 1996), an illness (Fassin, 2001; Rapp, 1999; Ticktin, 2008; Whyte, 2009), or physical damage (Petryna, 2002)—but because they wish to withdraw their children from an intervention that would change their bodies. These groups seek to affirm the legitimacy of bodies considered abnormal even in the absence of any diagnosis or illness. In Italy, indeed, normal bodies are vaccinated bodies, and non-vaccinated bodies are deviations from the standard. Parents who do not want their children to be vaccinated therefore form a minority that claims the right to give citizenship to 'abnormal' bodies.

Another peculiar feature of parental groups is that they are a form of biosociality by proxy: their members campaign for the biological rights of their children, not for their own bodies. Their advocacy arises not only from their close connection to their children, but also as a way to affirm and defend their own position as good parents in society. By fighting to raise awareness about the potential risks of vaccination (and thus, they believe, saving lives), they also seek to have parents who do not vaccinate their children recognized as good and responsible parents despite (or because of) their choice. In recent decades in the Global North, 'proper' parenting has assumed huge political importance (Faircloth and Lee, 2010), and the meaning of parental responsibility has shifted from parental authority to parental accountability (Reece, 2006). In this climate, the political activities of parental groups are driven not only by a humanitarian goal (save lives), an enlightened mentality (disseminate alternative knowledge), or an indi- vidualistic need (avoid vaccination for their children), but also—and most importantly—by an endeavour to gain legitimacy as parents. Vaccination choice is thus linked to the social recognition of specific social identities.

Italian parents can avoid vaccinating their children simply by paying a fine of around €240. In six regions (Veneto, Lombardy, Piedmont, Tuscany, Sardinia, Emilia-Romagna, and Trentino) out of 20, paediatric vaccina- tions are still compulsory but parents are exempted from paying the fine. Therefore, parents who merely wish not to vaccinate their children have little reason to spend time and energy as members of parental groups. In the province of Trento there were 5454 newborns in 2010, of which 209 were not vaccinated,[1] equivalent to 3.8% of all newborns. Vaccinareinformati, the

---

1   Data were kindly disclosed to the researcher by the Preventive Medicine Service of Trento Province.

local parental group, has only around 200 members. The coordinator told me that about 5000 people had asked for information since the foundation of the parental group, but only a few of them had formally joined the organization and participated actively in its meetings and other activities.

Belonging to a parental group thus entails more than simply avoiding vaccination; it is a political and institutional practice. Since the beginning, Vaccinareinformati organized campaigns to bring public and institutional attention to the matter of vaccination, and it has achieved some level of success in that in Trentino parents are now exempted from paying a fine if they choose not to vaccinate their children. When the fine was still being administered, the group advised its members to not pay the fine immediately, but rather to undertake a fairly complex medical and legal process in order to emphasize the meaning of their choice and attract attention. Parents had to first request a meeting with a medical professional at the local public health board, during which they raised their concerns about vaccines, often relying on information and questions published on the Vaccinareinformati website. If the parents and the medical professional did not reach an agreement by the end of the meeting, the parents were asked to assume responsibility for not vaccinating their children by signing a self-discharge form. The form stated that the parents were fully informed about the risks and released doctors from any liability. Vaccinareinformati recommended that parents not sign the form but instead declare that they had not received enough information. In this manner, they hoped to highlight the gaps in the communication of possible risks and the inadequacy of the current adverse reaction tracking system.

Since 2012, Trentino parents who do not vaccinate their children do not have had to pay a fine. Before 2012, parental group members also campaigned on legal grounds, claiming that vaccination enforcement contravenes Article 32 of the Italian Constitution, which states: 'Nobody can be obliged to receive a specific medical treatment unless provided by law. The law cannot, in any case, violate the limits imposed with respect of the person'. Vaccinareinformati advised parents not to pay the fine but instead to send a letter to the regional health board, using a form letter that could be downloaded from their website. In this letter, parents declared that they had not received sufficient information and emphasized contradictions and omissions in the vaccination enforcement policy. After submitting such a letter, families were invited to meet with the regional coordinator of health; among the families I followed, this invitation came anywhere from a few months up to five years later. If no agreement was reached on this occasion either, parents were advised to refer their case to a justice of the peace. The recent exemption from the fine in case of opting out of vaccination is one of the first results, and it has been welcomed by the group's members. It can be concluded from the foregoing description that parental groups are socialities. Whether they are also *bio*socialities is more debatable, a question I will address in the remainder of the paper.

Following 'the normal course of nature'

When I first looked for information about vaccination, I talked to Maria, a representative from Vaccinareinformati. I told her about my doubts and fears associated with the idea of not having my daughter vaccinated. Very charmingly, Maria described all the growth and development advantages of non-vaccinated children by reporting the case of her own child and other cases:

> You can see, you will see yourself. Mattia [her non-vaccinated son], for example, started to walk much earlier than Sara [her vaccinated daughter]. At 10 months he was already walking, and coordination is much enhanced in children who haven't been vaccinated. I don't know, maybe these are just coincidences, but most parents report similar things. And you'll see, when your daughter goes to kindergarten she'll maybe get sick often and more easily, but the illness will be much milder and recovery much quicker. These children are just stronger. And at school, you'll see that they can read earlier than their peers. Overall, they're more, I don't know, they are more vital. It's obvious. If you don't touch the organism, if you let it *follow the normal course of nature*, you'll have lots of advantages. (Emphasis added)[2]

Maria defined the 'normal course of nature' as the gold standard for children's growth. According to her, if organisms are not 'touched' by vaccines, their bodies can express their original potential to a greater extent.

If in Italy normal bodies are vaccinated bodies and abnormal bodies are non-vaccinated ones, for parental groups the terms of the argument are reversed. This inversion has important theoretical and political implications. For mainstream Italian parents, the reference point of a body's normality is compliance with an institutional regime of care, while for the members

---

2   The interview excerpts included in this article were all translated by the author from Italian to English.

of parental groups this reference point is the capacity of the body to adapt flexibly to any situation and to express its original potential. In Georges Canguilhem's (1989) words, the first is a *normal* body (one normalized by sociopolitical standards); the latter is a *normative* body. As Monica Greco (2004, p. 3) points out, '"normativity" refers to a capacity to institute, or to be the source of norms'. From this perspective, health is the body's capacity to adapt dynamically to any given situation.

According to parents critical of vaccinations, this potential for dynamic adaptation is diminished in vaccinated bodies. Sofia, a young mother whose child had not been vaccinated, told me:

> Of course I'm afraid that my decision [not to vaccinate] may be wrong. Can you imagine if Anna died because of tetanus or meningitis? I mean, I would be destroyed. It would be as if I'd killed her. I can't even think about that. Look, I've got the shivers just thinking about it. But then I look at the risks of vaccination, which are more frequent than we think, you just have to look around today. [I interviewed her at a parental group meeting where a number of disabled children were present.] And all the long-term effects—so many cancers, leukaemias, mental disorders—there must be an explanation somewhere. But what convinces me most is that we're heading towards a very uncertain future. Antibiotic-resistant diseases are increasing, and things like that, strange epidemics. [pauses] I mean, Anna will be fitter to fight them, for which there'll be no medications, maybe, because her organism hasn't been spoiled by the vaccine and so her immune system will be stronger. [pause] Yes, I accept these risks as an investment in her future.

According to Sofia, it is better to have a strong organism able to adapt to different conditions than to be well protected against a few select diseases but with a weak and inflexible immune system. She was aware that not vaccinating has its risks, and that it is emotionally difficult to handle. At the same time, she was compelled by the notion that we are 'heading for a very uncertain future'. Intervening in the body's physiology to prevent only a few and rare diseases (those covered by vaccinations) is seen as limiting bodily capacities, which is a danger, given the unpredictability of how diseases might change in the future. According to Sofia, taking risks by not vaccinating is acceptable if the body is better able to deal with the unexpected.

This logic unsettles the very theoretical basis of the concept of biosociality, introduced in sociological and anthropological debates to emphasize

how culture has absorbed nature in a biotechnological age. The normativity expressed in these parental descriptions of a healthy body counters
the postmodern argument that normativity (an organic regime) is now
normality (a sociocultural regime). Rose (2001, pp. 19–20), in reflecting upon
Canguilhem, affirms that 'normativity no longer can be understood in terms
of the self-regulation of a vital order—if it ever was. Normativity now [in
postmodern thought] becomes a matter of normality, of social and moral
judgments about whether particular lives are worth living'. In contrast to
postmodern understandings of the body, parental groups meet in name
of the primacy of the organic over culture, of normativity over normality.

A healthy body is, according to parental groups, one that is truthful to a
vital order. This understanding resonates with Canguilhem's (1989, p. 100)
distinction between *organic* and *social* normality/normativity as overlap-
ping domains in which, the organic has autonomy and logical priority over
culture because the sociocultural norm 'cannot impose on life just those
ways whose mechanism is intelligible to it'. The organic, as depicted by the
parents of this study, is very different from essentialist ideas of 'nature': it
is not a static, bounded and pre-established concept. For example, Maria
said that a healthy body is one that 'follow[s] the course of nature'. Using
the verb 'follow' and the word 'course', this phrase expresses well how she
makes sense of nature: not as a thing, but a dynamic process with autonomy
and generative power.

Bios versus *zoē*

To better unravel the implications of these parents' understanding of nature
as a vital order, it may be helpful to consider Giorgio Agamben's (1998)
reflections on the terms '*bios*' and '*zoē*'. Agamben (1998, pp. 1–3) illustrates
how, at the time of ancient Greeks, *bios* was just one of the possible ways
to refer to life. For Aristotle, '*bios*' meant the life of human beings: the life
lived among other people in the polis. The famous definition of man as
a 'political animal' stressed the fact that man's original animality was
crucially shaped by his propensity for political life. *Zoē*, in contrast, was
life of any existing being: all organic life in opposition to non-living death.
It was defined as biological life at its minimum, subsistence, and devoid
of any political implication; it could be lived to its fullest even in the wild
outside the polis.

Zoē, which Agamben also calls 'bare life', is very similar to the idea of
organic life advanced by parental-group members: they want bodies to

be left free to deploy their physiological potential, 'following the course of nature', without human interference. Vaccinated bodies, by contrast, are not *zoē* anymore, because they have been modified their original physiology through medical intervention. They are now normal, not normative.

Is 'zoēsocialities' perhaps a better term for characterizing the sociality formed by parental groups? While this term captures the specific claim advanced by parental groups, my aim is not simply to add a new term to the already bourgeoning literature on socialites related to biological conditions. Instead, I wish to shed light on a neglected dimension of health and vital processes: indeterminacy (Greco, 2004). Parents critical of vaccinations speak about health's indeterminacy, and not in a negative and deprived sense, as lack of something. Rather, in their conceptualization, health is a state that can be defined by—but is not limited to—biomedical interpretations and interventions. This understanding thus expands the ontological and epistemological reach of the concept of health.

Greco (2004, p. 10) writes of a 'vital order' that 'encompasses but exceeds both human consciousness and knowledge. [...] It refers to an order of possibility that includes the social and much more besides.' From this perspective, the order of the biological cannot simply be conflated with the order of the sociocultural, as the former exceeds the latter. Biology is not determined in its entirety by our scientific knowledge and technology. Some biological conditions—such as not being vaccinated—can be relevant to life exactly because of their indeterminacy. In order to recognize the importance of vital—and indeterminate—processes, Greco proposes to extend political recognition to them. This is what parents of non-vaccinated children argue for: a reclamation of citizenship for bare life on its own terms, not in a reductive assimilation to a standard.

Agamben (1998, pp. 71–111) illustrates how, in ancient times, bare life was considered an exception. But bare life was at the core of political life because the act itself of banning it generated the possibility for political life. The value of bare life was found in its being the dialectical prerequisite for politics. Agamben's (1998, p. 13) provocative question—'Does *zoē* really need to be politicized, or is politics not already contained in *zoē* as its most precious center?'—can be interpreted as an invitation to reverse the gaze, as parents critical of vaccination do, and to consider bare life as political in its own terms, no longer just an abstract limit point or rhetorical horizon.

Conclusion

In most scholarly discussions, biosocialities are seen to emerge from biomedical diagnoses of physiological conditions. This chapter suggests that socialities may develop beyond biomedicine and around contested understandings of health. This perspective has political consequences. When I first discussed biosociality with a friend, he immediately reacted by saying, 'But [biosociality] is a paradox: what is biological is biological, what is social is social!' Scholars arguing for the isomorphism between culture and nature might have a concern opposite to that voiced by my friend, seeing the term 'biosociality' more as a tautology. Quite rightly, they might ask: How can the biological not be social at the same time? Can the biological in any way escape its political rootedness? And can sociality be fleshless?

These are reasonable questions, and in many cases the term 'biosociality' can be considered a tautology. The case of parents critical of vaccination adds to this debate the consideration that the term 'biosociality' can never be a metonymy (a part (culture) as a name for the whole (bios)), as, according to these parents, the organic is an autonomous dimension, yet one that sometimes overlaps with the social. The biological should not merely be understood as a biomedical norm, but as an organic normativity with a potential that exceeds cultural determination and constitution. Parents critical of vaccination assemble beyond both biomedical or cultural determinations of 'nature'. Their sociality acquires a meaning by affirming the indeterminacy of nature, and defining a healthy body as one able to adapt to any given condition. This adaptation is dynamic and caught up in always surprising (Daston and Prak, 1998) and manifold ways.

The sociality of these parents shows that neither biomedical definitions nor techno-cultural crafting of nature exhaust life's potentiality. 'Flattening nature onto politics' (Greco, 2004, p. 12) comes with a cost: it excludes nature (in the sense defined above) from speculation and from politics as a legitimate order of possibility. Anti-vaccination parental groups are a salutary challenge in this regard because they bring attention to the political value of health as indeterminacy and *potentia*. As Franklin et al. (2009, p. 9) have noted, 'nature and culture have become increasingly isomorphic while remaining distinct'; it is by continuing to debate the terms of this ongoing differentiation that novel ideas and perspectives may arise.

References

Agamben, G. (1998). *Homo sacer: Sovereign power and bare life.* Stanford: Stanford University Press.

Benatti, C., Ambrosi, F., and Rosa, C. (2006). *Vaccinazioni tra scienza e propaganda: Elementi critici di riflessione.* Turin: Il Leone Verde.

Canguilhem, G. (1989). *The normal and the pathological.* New York: Zone Books.

Daston, L., and Prak, K. (1998). *Wonders and the order of nature.* New York: Zone Books.

Faircloth C., and Lee, E. (2010). Introduction: 'Changing parenting culture'. *Sociological Research Online, 15*(4), 1.

Fassin, D. (2001). The biopolitics of otherness: Undocumented foreigners and racial discrimination in French public debate. *Anthropology Today, 17*(1), 3–7.

Franklin, S., Lury, C., and Stacey, J. (2000). *Global Nature, Global Culture.* New York: SAGE Publications

Gava, R. (2008). *Le vaccinazioni pediatriche: Revisione delle conoscenze scientifiche.* Padua, Italy: Salus Infirmorum.

Greco, M. (2004). The politics of indeterminacy and the right to health. *Theory, Culture & Society, 21*(6), 1–22.

Haraway, D. (1997). *Modest witness.* New York: Routledge.

Lock, M., and Nguyen, V.-K. (2010). *An anthropology of biomedicine.* London: Wiley-Blackwell.

Martin, J., and Marshall, F.J. (2003). New tendencies and strategies in international immunisation: GAVI and The Vaccine Fund. *Vaccine, 21*(7–8), 587–592.

Moulin, A.M. (1991). *Le dernier langage de la médecine: Historie de l'immunologie de Pasteur au Sida.* Paris: Presses Universitaires de France.

Petryna, A. (2002). *Life exposed: Biological citizens after Chernobyl.* Princeton: Princeton University Press.

Poland, G.A., and Jacobson, R.M. (2001). Understanding those who do not understand: A brief review of the anti-vaccine movement. *Vaccine, 19*(17–19), 2440–2445.

Rabinow, P. (1992). Artificiality and enlightenment: From sociobiology to biosociality. In J. Crary and S. Kwinter, eds., *Incorporations* (pp. 234–252). New York: Urzone.

Rabinow, P. (1996). *Essays on the anthropology of reason.* Princeton: Princeton University Press.

Raffaetà, R. (2012). When 'to choose' is 'to care': The case of paediatric vaccinations. *Suomen Antropologi: Journal of the Finnish Anthropological Society, 37*(3), 8–23.

Rapp, R. (1999). *Testing women, testing the fetus: The social impact of amniocentesis in America.* New York: Routledge.

Reece, H. (2006). From parental responsibility to parenting responsibly. In M. Freeman, ed., *Law and sociology* (pp. 459–473). Oxford: Oxford University Press.

Rose, N. (2001). The politics of life itself. *Theory, Culture & Society, 18*, 1–30.

Serravalle, E. (2009). *Bambini super-vaccinati: Saperne di più per una scelta responsabile.* Turin: Il Leone Verde.

Strathern, M. (1992). *After nature: English kinship in the late twentieth century.* Cambridge: Cambridge University Press.

Ticktin, M. (2008). *Causalities of care.* Berkeley: University of California Press.

Whyte, S.R. (2009). Health identities and subjectivities. *Medical Anthropology Quarterly, 23*(1), 6–15.

2 Emerging animistic socialities?

An example of transnational appropriation of curanderismo[1]

Franz Graf

While for some scholars 'sociality' is an explicitly 'human capacity for the social' (Barnard and Spencer, 1996, p. 622), relational approaches have received increasing attention for their promise in overcoming a nature–culture dichotomy by considering all phenomena 'social' if they are 'intrinsically interactive' (Cook et al., quoted in Long and Moore, 2013, p. 13). '[A]ll life would be social life', argues Ingold (1997, p. 249), refusing to distinguish between human and nonhuman sociality. Although Long and Moore (2013, p. 13) have little doubt that we live in a relational world, they warn that relational views 'all too quickly conflate ontological interventions with cryptonormative programmes of how we, as analysts and subjects, should engage with a relational world'. The question is, in what ways do people engage with this relationality, something that is 'always informed by historically and spatially particular practices of ethical imagination' (Long and Moore, 2013, p. 14)?

The ethnographic research underlying this paper was conducted with people in Mexico, England, Germany, and Austria who share an interest in magico-therapeutic ways of becoming 'healthy' and producing 'health', and who engage in apprenticeships in groups led by a *curandera* (practitioner of Latin American folk medicine) (Graf, 2009, 2013).[2] This field of social actors is characterized by a strong desire to push and transform their own concepts of 'sociality' ('real-world sociality') in 'new directions' (see Long and Moore, 2013, p. 3)—and, in particular, in animistic directions. According to Whyte (2009, p. 7), the allegiance to one particular medical subsystem can be seen as 'a kind of medicinal cultural politics that places a person by expressing loyalty to one system in opposition to another'.

1   I thank Gertraud Seiser for helping me to think through some of the issues presented here. I would also like to express my gratitude to Bernhard Hadolt and Elke Mader for constructive criticism and feedback. I am also grateful to Robert Mixan and Dominic Rooney for their valuable comments on an earlier version of the manuscript.
2   What I refer to here as the European appropriation of *curanderismo* can be academically framed under the term 'neo-Shamanisms' (see Wallis, 2003), which now constitute a part of complementary and alternative medicine (CAM) (Reece, 2010).

I argue that the emerging sociality in question combines practical, cosmologically embedded applications for the production of 'health' or 'balance' and a theory of a 'good and healthy way of living', which is opposed to diagnosed 'ills of modernity'. *Curanderismo* in Europe (and urban Mexico) attracts practitioners because it promises an alternative to modern Western thought and addresses desires to overcome desacralized, individualistic, and alienated relations. This contribution seeks to answer the following questions: Which academic trends accompany the creation of new animistic socialities? What are the historical and political contexts in which *curanderismo* is appropriated by European practitioners? Which ethical models and explanations attract them? Which practices are part of these discourses and which meanings are being negotiated? What desires of European recipients are being addressed, and how are the aspirations to be contextualized in recent diagnoses of our postmodern, precarious work society and its deprivations?

Some remarks towards the revaluation of 'animism'

'Animism,' defined as 'a belief in souls or spirits', is one of the oldest anthropological concepts (Bird-David, 1999, p. 68). It was introduced during European colonization in the nineteenth century by Edward B. Tylor to designate 'original', 'primitive' religions (Prufer, 2006, p. 79). People who perceive objects and non-human entities as animate by attributing to them an interiority or individual characteristics were described as animistic (see Tylor, 1913 [1871]). Tylor understood animism as the superstitious and erroneous attribution of life, soul, and spirit to inanimate objects of nature, which he saw as the lowest rung on a hierarchical model of religions. Believers would project life where there is none (for example, in stones, deceased persons, clouds), in other words attributing non-human things with human characteristics such as intentionality, agency, and subjective character. Tylor wrote his text as an explicit polemic for 'the furtherance of rationalism against the mistakes of religious belief' (Harvey, 2010, p. 15). In his evolutionary history of religion, Tylor drew the development of man from animism, polytheism, and monotheism all the way to modern science. This 'old' animism was constituted as a negative mirror image for the project of modernity. The concept of erroneous animation of inanimate objects was formed on the basis of a dichotomy between 'spiritual and materialistic' or 'society and nature' accompanied by the belief in Western science's monopoly on truth about the world (Bird-David, 1999, p. 68; see Lewis,

1994). Povinelli (1995, pp. 505f.), drawing on Baudrillard, notes: 'subaltern perspectives on [...] the nature of human–environment interactions are subordinate to the dominant perspective not only because they are popularly imagined as preceding it in social evolutionary time but also because they are represented as beliefs rather than a method for ascertaining truth'. Thus, from a modern Western perspective, 'the animists' were considered to be cognitively undeveloped and to have a childish and flawed view of the world.

Anthropological analysis now largely acknowledges diverse entities as 'fellow participants in the same world' that 'co-constitute each others' environments' (Long and Moore, 2013, p. 13). However, modern Western thought and science, which Descola (2013 [2006], p. 84) correlates with the 'ontology of naturalism', identify an anomic and unified 'Nature' devoid of interiority that is contrasted with a multiplicity of human cultures endowed with 'mind, the soul, subjectivity, a moral conscience, language and so forth'. In terms of the corresponding socialities, Descola (2013 [2006], p. 86) argues that '[a] nimism is extremely liberal in its attribution of sociality to non-humans, while naturalism reserves the privilege of it to everything that is not deemed natural'. Scholars such as Nurit Bird-David, Philippe Descola, Tim Ingold, Eduardo Viveiros de Castro, and Graham Harvey have contributed in the past two decades to a reassessment of the concept of animism. The ontology of animism, following Ingold (2006, p. 10), is not a way of thinking *about* the world but of being alive *to* it, 'characterised by a heightened sensitivity and responsiveness, in perception and action, to an environment that is always in flux, never the same from one moment to the next'. According to Harvey (2005, p. xvii), animisms are 'theories, discourses and practices of relationship, of living well, of realizing more fully what it means to be a person, and a human person, in the company of other persons, not all of whom are human but all of whom are worthy of respect'. Here, animism is understood in terms of its relationality, and its potential to revaluate the boundaries between life and non-life, nature and culture, subjectivity and objectivity. Moreover, animism becomes a moral issue, one that addresses questions of 'the good life'. Such approaches to animism could be understood as transference of the scientists' desires, motivated by a search for 'other' socialities that ought to provide the 'better life' for their members (Adler, 1993, p. xxi). However, I would argue that there is still something to gain from an alternative analysis: the reinterpretation of animism and relational critique in the research and work of Irving A. Hallowell (2002 [1960]).

Hallowell studied the Ojibwa people in southern Canada and found that within the Algonquian language, there is a difference between animate and inanimate gender: a suffix on a noun indicates whether it refers to animate persons or inanimate objects. Hallowell coined the phrase 'other-than-human person'. Thus the term 'person' is not equated with humans; it is a large concept, covering all creatures that communicate intentionally and behave relationally to others. The Ojibwa share the world with a variety of relational persons (tree people, fish people, bird people, stone people) and the question for them 'is not "how do we know stones are alive?" but "what is the appropriate way for people, of any kind, to relate?"' (Harvey, 2010, p. 20). Personhood in this sense is not understood as the intrinsic attribute of an individual, but represents a 'becoming' and a 'being alive' through an entanglement in a particular relationship (Ingold, 2000, p. 97). Unlike Tylor, Hallowell does not speak of a 'belief system', but of a 'world view', a relational way of being in the world. He relocates 'the religious in the actual relationships which constitute the everyday world' (Morrison, 2000, p. 35). Thus, relationships are seen as a matter of responsibility between humans and other animals, plants, and even cosmic beings who share the same world and have socio-religious motives towards each other (Morrison, 2000, p. 23ff.; see also Viveiros de Castro, 1998). This revaluation of animism and the project of 'new animism' with its moral implications could be interpreted as a welcome support in the study of the emerging socialities of practitioners, and their active engagement with epistemologies and ontologies that differ from those of the dominant societies in which they live (see Rountree, 2012, p. 317). The following section considers some of the historical and political contexts in which new animistic socialities emerge.

Contexts of appropriation from Mexico to Europe

Curanderismo (from Spanish '*curar*', which means to cure/to heal) is used as a generic term for a wide range of ideas and practices concerning the production of health in Latin America, ranging from simple home remedies to spiritual operations. According to a practitioner in London, *curanderismo* comes from a whole big melting pot of indigenous 'medicines [and] has roots in Africa, it has roots in Europe, as well as the North and South Americas and Mexico' (see also Mull and Mull, 1983). *Curanderos/as* can be compared with *yerberos* (experts of medicinal herbs), *parteras* (midwives), and *sobadores* (masseuses) and are distinguished by the fact that they work both with the 'physical' as well as with the 'supernatural world'[3] (Trotter and Chavira,

---

3   It is usual in the anthropological literature to subsume the fields of activity of *curanderos/ as* under the generic term 'shamanism' (see Saladin d'Anglure, 1996, p. 505).

1997, p. 9). The dichotomy of nature and super-nature, as well as the idea of separation between physical and mental or physical and social dimensions, is within *curanderismo* far less common than in Western modes of thought (Mull and Mull, 1983, p. 734; Trotter and Chavira, 1997, p. 14f.; Nigenda et al., 2001, p. 11). According to a *curandera* in Mexico with whom I worked, this is due to the indigenous perspective of the cosmos: 'Although it consists of two halves, two forces or energies, the focus lies not on the separation and distinction but on the relationship between the two dimensions.' If this relationship is not in balance, disease will arise (see Viesca, 1997, p. 164). An imbalance in the sense of 'too much' or 'too little' can express itself in manifold ways—physical, psychological, mental, social, or spiritual.[4]

While indigenous local knowledge has been marginalized by modernization, it could be suggested that since the 1980s revitalization movements have arisen (see Vitebsky, 2003). In response to the crises of industrial development and modern ideologies of progress, urban forms of traditional knowledge have been developed (Hoppál, 2007, p. vii f.; Berenzon-Gorn et al., 2006). The shaman (or *curandera/o*) became a symbol for indigenous resistance against (neo)colonial powers and Western hegemonic world views (DuBois, 2011, p. 109). Through mediating cultural knowledge and the formation of cultural identities he or she plays a significant role in a 'social healing' process (Hoppál, 1992, p. 199). In the Valley of Mexico, in the region at the northern edge of the megalopolis of Mexico City, a place deeply affected by suburbanization, indigenous knowledge and local treatment methods are being revived and implemented within urban and semi-urban settings. The Mexican 'school' for *curanderismo* in whose transnational 'community of practice' (Lave and Wenger, 1991) I studied and conducted ethnographic field research from 2004 to 2007 was founded in the mid-1990s by Gabriela, a *curandera* and traditional teacher. She became fascinated with the knowledge and practices in her rural communities as a young teenager and learned from and worked with local healers. Along the way, especially in her urban school and university environment, her indigenous appearance (rural dialect, darker skin, clothing, hairstyle) and also her interest in 'Mexican traditions' were devaluated and she experienced discrimination. It is this experience of being discriminated against that stimulated her 'struggle for recognition' (Whyte, 2009, p. 7) of indigenous practices, cosmologies, and identities. Becoming a healer and traditional teacher in her village provided her with an adequate social role to negotiate

---

4   The variety of used methods in *curanderismo* reflects and addresses these layers (Graf, 2009).

the difference between the 'two cultures' described by Frye (1996, p. 9): 'In the colonial era these two cultures were known as Indian and Spanish. Today (and even then) it would perhaps be more accurate to speak instead of rural and urban cultures.'

Gabriela's 'medical centre' is a base for the distribution of knowledge, practices, and political ideologies, and consists of several areas. There is the waiting room, with anatomy atlases adorning the walls, *ranchera* background music, and an assistant (her sister) who measures the waiting patients' blood pressure and fills out their medical history forms. The *curanderas* treat the patients from the village, the region, the adjacent city, and even other states in two small treatment rooms. There is Nahuatl art on the walls, mats on the floor, and towels, oils, and creams ready for the massages. The altar utensils, rattles and flutes, lotions, and other paraphernalia are ready for ritualistic use. One room is filled with remedies; this is where the Mexican and Peruvian herbs, tinctures, and essences are processed and compiled for the patients. Two days a week the medical centre is open for patients and is heavily frequented. Through observation and assistance, students learn directly while practicing with more experienced practitioners. One day a week is reserved for lectures and talks, during which Gabriela draws on the philosophical, historical, and ideological backgrounds of her *curanderismo*. Teaching the healing methods to the group usually takes place on weekends in the form of workshops. This phenomenon of a 'school for healers' is difficult to understand in 'either-or' perceptions of traditional, urban, or neo-shamanic practices.[5] Both rural Mexicans (who emphasize their traditional roots) and, increasingly, urban Mexicans (in search of an indigenous identity) turn to medical experts in rural areas; they are joined by people from the United States and Europe (who are looking for alternative ways of dealing with illness and health) in making use of *curanderismo*.

Recently the *curandera* has tried to secure her field of activity within the scenario of globalization (cf. Mader, 2004, p. 8). Gabriela travels to Europe and the United States; while she is away, more advanced students take care of the patients at her centre in Mexico. The help of a Viennese medical anthropologist (her first European student) and Gabriela's dual educational background (both 'Western' urban socialization and a 'traditional')

---

5   These categories often contribute to an inaccurate assessment of practitioners and direct academic attention to certain phenomena and not to others. The designation of shamans as 'original', 'authentic', or 'real' is according to Wallis (2003, p. 50), a Western imposition, which partly arises from a misguided search for a single primordial shamanism and ignores 'the agentic urbanisation of shamanisms in many places which cannot be regarded as less authentic or valid'.

rural background), allow her to negotiate different realities in different localities. In England, Austria, and Germany she offers treatments and holds lectures and seminars on 'Medicine and Philosophy'. Practitioners from diverse backgrounds—psychotherapists, physiotherapists, 'Heilpraktiker' (naturopathic practitioners), biomedical doctors, and artists—attend the seminars and learn about alternative approaches to handling illness and health apart from the biomedical mainstream. They often draw from a wide range of more common 'esoteric' ideas and practices to render *curanderismo* intelligible.[6] According to Jakobsen (summarized in Reece, 2010, p. 9), the gravitational force towards neo-shamanisms is due to a stress caused by 'having spiritual experiences in an increasingly materialistic and desacralized society', which cannot provide a basis for the meaningful integration of these experiences. The ethical imagination effective in *curanderismo*—the capacity for 'endowing things of the imagination and the mind with meaning and significance' (Moore, 2013, p. 38)—revaluates these experiences as an indication of 'the gift of the healer' (*el don*). Something that has estranged practitioners in one system of thought becomes a resource for identity in another. Hundreds of people in Europe have come in contact with the group, but only a few engage with the hierarchical education system and commit to the time-consuming and resource-intensive training. Those that do regularly travel to Mexico, pursue self-study, practice in the group, and organize workshops for the travelling *curanderas*. Since 2003 fewer than 20 apprentices have completed their training in this particular school and built their livelihood on the practice.[7] Some of them are teaching their own students in *curanderismo* and are in close contact with Gabriela's Mexican 'headquarters'. Others have tried to patent the medicine under German law and have been cast out from the community. The following section will elaborate on some ideas and practices that are constitutive of the identities of practitioners and their ethical imagination.

6   Emerging animistic socialities are deeply affected by Western esoteric traditions (Von Stuckrad, 2002, 2003) and practices such as shiatsu, taijiquan, qigong, acupuncture, neo-shamanisms, wilderness therapy, etc.; there is a momentum here that calls for further research but that cannot be considered in this contribution.

7   To make sense of the low numbers of practitioners in Europe, the legal situations in each country need to be considered. While in England—still the most successful place for *curanderas/ os*—a neoliberal health market seems to contribute to self-assured application, a repressive paragraph (§ 184 'Kurpfuscherei') in the Austrian criminal code (StGB-AT) prohibits the professional treatment of 'patients' by all but biomedical personnel.

Ethical models of socio-cosmic relationality

> I answer a phone call from Gabriela. She is on one of her working trips
> to England. We chat a bit and I cannot hold back my questions about her
> understanding of '*nahui ollin teotl*', the system of coordination which
> organizes the cosmos in four directions, '*cuatro movimiento*', as she
> translates it from Nahuatl: 'Are those forces intelligible as persons, as
> other-than-human persons?' 'No!' she replies vehemently and explains:
> 'That is a widespread confusion. For example "quezalcoatl", which we
> acknowledge in rituals when we face east is neither a god nor a person; it
> is a force, the essence of a beginning, it is light and logic, and it permeates
> all life, like the rising of the sun in the morning. We and everything that
> exists, everything that is alive, all persons, like the sun, the wind, the
> plants, the animals and the dead people, all are part of these processes
> of life.' (Field notes, May 2012)

During the training, models, explanations, and mythologies are mostly
transmitted through talks and stories and not in phone conversations. They
are performed in the presence of those forces and energies visualized in the
altar of the healer rather than simply narrated. The altar represents and is
the cosmos in which those narrative performances hold their truth; it is a
condensed model that ties the human to 'Father Sun', 'Mother Earth', the
directions, and other-than-human entities. An underlying idea of the stories
and explanations can be compared with that of Ojibwa ontology, where all
persons, whether human or not, have an overarching commonality. This
basis consists, in Hallowell's (2002 [1960], p. 41) words, of 'an inner vital
part that is enduring and an outward form which can change'. Sentience,
volition, memory, and speech are attributes of the inner essence and any
'thing' that possesses these attributes can become a person (Ingold, 2000,
p. 92). In the 'school' for *curanderismo* this principle is called 'four energies in
movement', which are said to permeate all life. Although European students
and anthropologists may make the mistake of confusing essences with
other-than-human persons, they are pressed to study the concept of 'respect'
that is integral to the relationship with either: 'Respect your grandparents,
respect your parents, respect all beings and everything that exists so that
you live in harmony with your surroundings.' This precept, one of the first
revealed to the adepts, extends beyond a Christian notion of charity and
implies the imperative to respect all life (not just human life). In this ethical
imagination respectful and responsible actions within moralized socio-
cosmic frameworks are not matters of free decision. They are a necessity for

the production of 'health' or 'balance' and need to be constantly embodied through relational practices. While novices learn the practical skills of a trade, the learning processes are also concerned with the creation of moral sensibilities, cultural identities, and selves (Dilley, 2001, p. 606). According to Whyte (2009, p. 7), social identity is about the revaluation of difference and similarity between others and selves and is often defined through what it rejects and what it renders as its exterior. The identity politics at stake oppose desacralized notions of life, in which nature and the cosmos are rendered inanimate, devoid of any interiority, separated from moral commitment, and open to objectified and abstract analysis. Reification and commodification of relations between humans and the earth are projected as inhuman concepts that lack the knowledge about the interrelatedness of life and thereby cause imbalances—consciously or unconsciously. This ethical imagination and the employed identity politics could be seen as a need to 'fight the windmills' of biopower that 'brought life and its mechanisms into the realm of explicit calculations' (Foucault, quoted in Inda, 2005, p. 16).

A more-than-human community of practice

Students in *curanderismo* learn to address a variety of other-than-human agencies[8] and deal with them accordingly. As helpers, their impact, in addition to the *magnetismo* (power of attraction) of the healer and the willpower of the patient, is crucial for the success of a treatment. More than the control of 'spirits', it is a matter of knowledge, respect, and negotiation skills (cf. Hutton, 2001; Harvey, 2010). In their attempt to 'restore balance' *curanderas/os* continually develop those skills, for example, how to talk to medicinal plants and how to listen to them, how to ask the 'grandparents'[9] for their assistance, and how to establish social relationships that go beyond the boundaries of life and death. One *curandera* from London, who studied under Gabriela for seven years, asks the plants she uses in a healing session for help. She lovingly touches them, cordially calls them 'grandmothers', and talks to them. She asks them for advice and sees plants not only as phytotherapeutic drugs: 'You ask them for help because you can't do any healing on your own. This is the way I have learned to deal with the grandparents.'

---

8   While they can be seen as either the cause or the remedy for illness, because of lack of space, I shall just deal with their beneficial influences.

9   For a discussion of the term 'grandparent' and its use in relation to a variety of human and nonhuman persons, see Hallowell (2002 [1960]) and Wallis (2009).

Plants become friends and colleagues that may be met during a walk in the
woods; they are approached slowly, a relationship is established, and the
healers get to know them and learn to trust them.

'Grandparents' and other-than-human-persons are addressed in prayers
during treatments: 'Please take my hands, take my spirit, my mind, and my
body to help this patient.' A Viennese *curandera* reports that when her spiritual helper participates in a ritual she feels 'a deep trust spreading through
me, a confidence that I am not alone, but that there are other forces at work,
those who know more and are able to do more than myself.' The 65-year-old
healer from Salzburg also experiences support from a very good friend and
colleague who was herself a *curandera*, and who died five years ago. She still
accompanies her when she receives the people of the village in her treatment
room: 'I just look at the picture of her [...] and I say, please help me, because
I do not know everything. [...] I can feel her supportive power in the room.'
In return the healer regularly visits the grave of her friend and on occasion
brings flowers and food to thank her. The fellowship with non-humans plays
an important role in *curanderismo* and various agents are addressed as participants in an interdependent world with the capacity to produce effects.
Practitioners are enthusiastic about being part of a 'cosmic community', part
of a 'large family [...] with all that exists', stressing a relatedness and contact
between themselves and the world. The subordination under this ideology
is constantly negotiated in the training. Learning, practice, and the development of identity are interrelated aspects of the trajectories of apprentices,
especially in social groups that devote themselves to a collective practice
and share expert knowledge (Lave and Wenger, 1991). According to Long and
Moore (2013, p. 11), the generativity of ethical practice 'moulds the discursive
(and material) environments with which human beings engage', and 'indicates that one's own sociality, and the impulses that underpin it, might be at
least partly amenable to control'. In their aim to transform their real-world
sociality, practitioners stress the relevance of 'community' and respective
responsibilities. The individualism present in modern ideology is seen as 'vice'
that needs to be controlled. They attempt to balance a disequilibrium that is
thought to derive from an emphasis on competition instead of cooperation
and a 'sense of self' that is solely defined through human constituents.

Forces between bodies and materials

There is silence in the room; the *curandera* takes a few drops from a yellow
bottle, spreads it in her hands, holds them close to the patient's face and

says, 'Inhale, inhale deeply!' The 'perfume' triggers a slight cough. 'Be focused on anything that helps you! Connect with anything that makes you alive, anything that brings joy and happiness.' The *curandera* takes the flowers that have been drizzled with scented lotion by an assistant. She rubs and strikes the patient on all sides with the bunch. The patient begins to laugh, as the colourful buds, leaves and blossoms 'explode' on her body wrapped in white linen. Parts of the bunch spread throughout the room and form a 'blooming' circle on the floor around the patient, who stands in its centre with outstretched arms and closed eyes and is sighing slightly. A rich smell, a mixture of flowers, perfume, cotton, and more spreads through the room. Then the healer takes the raw eggs. Speaking the words, 'Can you imagine? These eggs are like little vacuum cleaners,' she scrubs the patient from head to toe, till the eggs start to 'totter'. 'Aha!' the healer reinforces this sound, 'can you hear how the eggs absorb the bad air?' With caution the assistant disposes of the eggs. (Field notes, May 2005)

In this description of a 'cleansing', or *limpia*, the patient is rubbed with scented lotions, flowers, and eggs to get rid of 'harmful vibrations' and to absorb 'healthy' ones. *Limpias* can also look quite different, and a variety of colourful, fragrant, sounding, and luminescent materials can be used. The patient's body is rubbed with flowers, herbs, candles, fruits, fire or water, rattles and feathers. In doing so there are two elements that are essential: Firstly, the invitation and drawing of forces that support, balance, strengthen, and help. This is done by the setting itself, through prayer, perfume, and touch. Secondly, all negative forces, all 'pathogenic vibrations' (such as anger, pain, *mal aire*), are blown away, cast out, rubbed off, and removed with the use of the aforementioned materials (see Wörrle, 2002; Trotter and Chavira, 1997). The patients can experience the treatment with all their senses: they hear the words of the healer and the sounds the things make when they touch the patients' bodies; they feel the rubbing and streaking; they smell the plants, lotions, and essences; they see the materials and colours that streak their clothes; and they sometimes feel relief and the presence of the numinous. In an explanatory model (Lewis, 1994) of this medicine, life is understood as a constant process of transformation embodied in all things. In this context the materials 'give themselves' to the patients; they die so that the patient can live. During the transformation, they 'give' their lives; their life force is taken through the treatment by the *curandera* in order to enhance the recipients' lives. The scattered and mashed remnants of the flowers and herbs and eggs, ready for the dung pile or dustbin, give testimony to the force of death that has been averted.[10] A proverb often used in the school is: 'Death so there is life and life so there is death.' This is negotiated by the *curandero/a* within the *limpia* between the bodies of the patients and the materials. In the sensual experience of the abovementioned transformation processes, the participants learn to negotiate the perspective of simultaneity of life and death, and the corresponding morals, alongside more common models of clear-cut boundaries and linear progression from one to the other. Bodies, things, and materials are entangled in a fragile equilibrium of a vital force (*ometeotl*) that has an impact on 'health'. The treatment is supposed to compensate for this instability; the awareness of the transformative bodily experience convinces practitioners of its reality. Modern perspectives of the individualized body as a closed, completed unit with clearly defined boundaries serve as a mirror image. The collective identity of practitioners is established in opposition to the idea that the body can be reduced to an objectifiable biological entity. The emphasis on transgressive, permeable, and fluid bodies and their senses (explicitly transcending body/mind dichotomies) seems to meet the need of practitioners for authentic and holistic experiences to oppose reification and alienation.

Concluding remarks

Faced with the contemporary world that is characterized by a 'loss of meaning' (Augé, 2011), demands for alternative approaches to situate human sociality in a more-than-human world are prevalent, both popularly and academically (see Hornborg, 2006, p. 28). In academia 'animism' has recently been theorized and revaluated in ontological terms. Scholars of the 'new' animism are rather astonished by 'being *in* the world' than by sociocultural 'belief' or 'knowledge' *about* the world. The perspectives developed thereby question the hegemony of the 'ontology of naturalism' (Descola, 2013 [2006]),

10   This raises questions about the exploitative appropriation of 'nature', which are in my opinion applicable to the 'New Age' end of the spectrum in the esoteric health market rather than the *curanderas* with whom I have worked. In the context of modern society, the non-human can easily be used as a pure resource for human enhancement without engaging in responsible and reciprocal relationships. A universalizing, romanticizing, and anthropomorphizing perspective on the non-human environment (as good, benign, and nurturing), integrated in a consumerist project-of-the-self, can provide a framework for its spiritual exploitation. 'Nature' becomes a rhetorical backdrop for the construction of identities and generates beliefs about it, instead of developing relational and respectful practices within it.

propose relational models with immanent moral implications (Harvey, 2005), and provide alternative concepts of 'personhood' that explicitly integrate 'non-humans' into a social realm (Hallowell, 2002 [1960]). Sociality is thus not defined as the *human* capacity to be social, but becomes a 'constitutive quality' of *all* relationships (Ingold, 2006, p. 190). However, it is hard not to agree with Long and Moore (2013, p. 13), who argue that social analysis has to question 'how and why that relationality is managed, directed and operationalized'. The ethical imagination and ethical practice are a core concern for ethnographic studies, not only in fields where social actors consciously try to transform the socialities they live by. The 'agency, motivation, intentionality, and desire', seen as the basis for 'personal and social transformation', need to be addressed in their spatial and historical contexts (Long and Moore, 2013, p. 11).

The ethical imagination of European *curanderas/os* can be contextualized in processes of revitalization and professionalization of *curanderismo* in Mexico. The involved identity politics provide discourses on the revaluation of indigenous knowledge and practices, and illuminate a dominant modern ontology. *Curanderismo*, as thought in Gabriela's 'school', combines on the one hand practical, cosmologically embedded applications for the production of 'health', and on the other hand a theory of a 'good and right way of living'. In summary, it can be said that *curanderismo* appeals to European practitioners because of their needs and desires for meaningful (respectful, communal, and embodied) relationships with a living world. The apprenticeship sensitizes and empowers them to engage in forms of direct relatedness and connectedness, sometimes neglected or taken for granted in the dominant world views in which they live. By means of social, situated learning (Lave and Wenger, 1991), students develop the practical skills of a craft, appropriate ideas and ideologies, and create a 'sense of self'. Seeing identity as 'a game of playing the vis-à-vis' (Whyte, 2009, p. 7), it could be suggested that it is an 'unhealthy modern ideology' that is characterized as desacralized, individualistic, and alienated, that practitioners wish to oppose.

How are the ethical imagination, the needs, and the desires of practitioners to be contextualized in recent diagnoses of the contemporary and its deprivations? Ethically infused modes of behaviour and their rationalization within socio-cosmic models support practitioners in their search for respectful and responsible actions (seen as the basis for an equilibrium within oneself, between others and the environing world). Could this desire for 'living a good and honourable life' be associated with the diagnosed social alienation in everyday consumer life? The reification of life processes and commodifying claims, the cultivation of false needs, and the desire for absolute control and perfect design seem to know no boundaries (Vaneigem, 2012 [1967]). The explanatory models are attractive to practitioners because they provide countervailing perspectives to 'objectifying' and 'mechanistic' viewpoints.

Moreover, *curanderas/os* have to develop relationships that 'transcend those which are maintained with human beings' (Hallowell, 2002 [1960]). Can the established subject positions, which situate them as participants in an interconnected world, be related to a diagnosed loss of community? The model of the individualized 'homo economicus' prefers competition rather than cooperation and shares a set of dichotomous constructs such as object/subject, nature/society, agency of humans/patiency of non-humans, personhood of humans/non-personhood of non-humans. These are constantly challenged by the subcultural practice of *curanderas/os*. The perspective on the human—as a 'cosmic being' who intimately shares the world with a variety of other beings, only some of whom are human—might answer a need to oppose a detachment from the world, with its concomitant illusion of total predictability and foreseeability (Ingold, 2000, p. 76).

Finally, I have pointed out that the healing methods of *curanderos/as* are experienced and perceived in the body, addressing a variety of senses. Could a need for bodily experiences of transformation be related to a diagnosed loss of the body? As the venue of a neoliberal world view, the body becomes an alienated consumer product; it is under pressure to be designed individually, to be manageable, and to be controllable (Schilling, 1993). The emphasis on the body and its senses (explicitly transcending body/mind dichotomies) seems to meet the need of practitioners for authentic and holistic experiences, and their desire to oppose alienation.

I have addressed the engagement with and in new animistic socialities and I am tempted to agree with Vitebsky (2003, p. 296) that local knowledge 'must always remain epistemologically marginal to global knowledge' as it takes on the 'fragmentary nature of the society by which it is appropriated'. However, the increasing scholarly attention to animism and its resonance with ethical imaginations and practices of social actors requires further research. In a process of 'othering' in new animistic socialities, social actors seem to identify with animistic subject positions (imagining relational morals) that are contrasts with naturalistic positions (imagined as objectified differentiation). While the 'old' animism served as a negative mirror image for the project of modernity, it is 'modernity' that serves as a negative mirror image for the project of the 'new' animism. Ethnographic studies on processes of meaning making in fields where people seek to alter the sociality by which they live, should bring interesting insights into the various ways of negotiating and reconciling conflicting socialities, epistemologies, and ontologies.

References

Adler, M. (1993). *Ethnopsychoanalyse: Das Unbewusste in Wissenschaft und Kultur*. Stuttgart: Schattauer.

Augé, M. (2011). *Nicht-Orte*. Munich: C.H. Beck.

Barnard, A., and Spencer, J. (1996). Sociality. In A. Barnard and J. Spencer, eds., *Encyclopedia of social and cultural anthropology* (p. 622). London: Routledge.

Berenzon-Gorn, S., Ito-Sugiyama, E., and Vargas-Guadarrama, A.L. (2006). Enfermedades y padereceres por los que se recurre a terapeutas tradicionales de la Ciudad de México. *Salud pública de México, 48*(1), 45–56.

Bird-David, N. (1999). 'Animism' revisited: Personhood, environment, and relational epistemology [and comments and reply]. *Current Anthropology, 40*(Suppl.), 67–91.

Descola, P. (2013). Beyond nature and culture. In G. Harvey, ed., *The handbook of contemporary animism* (pp. 77–91). Durham: Acumen. (Original work published in 2006.)

Dilley, R.M. (2001). Apprenticeship: Anthropological aspects. In N.J. Smelser, ed., *International encyclopedia of the social & behavioral sciences*. Amsterdam: Elsevier.

DuBois, T.A. (2011). Trends in contemporary research on shamanism. *Numen, 58*(1), 100–128.

Frye, D.L. (1996). *Indians into Mexicans: History and identity in a Mexican town*. Austin: University of Texas Press.

Graf, F. (2009). *Dicen por aquí, que una cosa es saber, otra cosa es hacer, otra cosa es sentir: Lehre in der mexikanischen Heilkunde am Beispiel der Gemeinschaft calpulli cencalli im Valle de México*. Unpublished master's thesis. Vienna University, Vienna, Austria.

Graf, F. (2013). 'Ich bin keine Mexikanerin, aber ich bin Mexica': Über die Aneignung einer mexikanischen Heilpraxis im Umfeld von Revitalisierung und internationaler Verbreitung. In V. Futterknecht, M. Kremser, and M. Noseck-Licul, eds., *Heilung in den Religionen* (pp. 467–483). Vienna: Lit-Verlag.

Hallowell, I.A. (2002). Ojibwa ontology, behavior, and world view. In G. Harvey, ed., *Readings in indigenous religions* (pp. 17–49). London: Bloomsbury. (Originally published in 1960.)

Harvey, G. (2005). *Animism: Respecting the living world*. London: Hurst & Co.

Harvey, G. (2010). Animism rather than shamanism: New approaches to what shamans do (for other animists). In B. Schmidt and L. Huskinson, eds., *Spirit possession and trance: New interdisciplinary perspectives* (pp. 14–34). London: Continuum.

Hoppál, M. (1992). Urban shamans: A cultural revival in the postmodern world. In A.-L. Siikala and M. Hoppál, eds., *Studies on shamanism* (pp. 197–209). Budapest: Akadémiai Kiadó.

Hoppál, M. (2007). *Shamans and traditions*. Budapest: Akadémiai Kiadó.

Hornborg, A. (2006). Animism, fetishism, and objectivism as strategies for knowing (or not knowing) the world. *Ethnos, 71*(1), 21–32.

Hutton, R. (2001). *Shamans: Siberian spirituality and the Western imagination*. New York: Bloomsbury Academic.

Inda, J.X. (2005). Analytics of the modern: An introduction. In J.X. Inda, ed., *Anthropologies of modernity: Foucault, governmentality, and life politics* (pp. 1–20). Oxford: Blackwell.

Ingold, T. (1997). Life beyond the edge of nature?: Or, the mirage of society. In J.D. Greenwood, ed., *The mark of the social: Discovery or invention?* (pp. 231–252). Lanham, MD: Rowman and Littlefield.

Ingold, T. (2000). *The perception of the environment: Essays in livelihood, dwelling and skill.* London: Routledge.

Ingold, T. (2006). Rethinking the animate, re-animating thought. *Ethnos, 71*(1), 9–20.

Lave, J., and Wenger, E. (1991). *Situated learning: Legitimate peripheral participation.* Cambridge: Cambridge University Press.

Lewis, G. (1994). Magic, religion and rationality of belief. In T. Ingold, ed., *Companion encyclopedia of anthropology* (pp. 563–590). London: Routledge.

Long, N.J., and Moore, H.L. (2013). Introduction: Sociality's new directions. In N.J. Long and H.L. Moore, eds., *Sociality: New directions* (pp. 1–24). New York: Berghahn Books.

Mader, E. (2004). Schamanismus. In *Kultur- und Sozialanthropologie Lateinamerikas: Eine Einführung* (6). Retrieved from the Lateinamerika-Studien Online website: http://www.lateinamerika-studien.at/content/kultur/ethnologie/ethnologie-354.html.

Moore, H.L. (2013). Avatars and robots: The imaginary present and the socialities of the inorganic. In N.J. Long and H.L. Moore, eds., *Sociality: New Directions* (pp. 25–41). New York: Berghahn Books.

Morrison, K. M. (2000). The cosmos as intersubjective: Native American other-than-human persons. In G. Harvey, ed., *Indigenous religions: A companion* (pp. 23–36). London: Cassell.

Mull, J.D., and Mull, D.S. (1983). A visit with a curandero. *The Journal of Western Medicine, 139*(5), 730–736.

Nigenda, G., Locket, L., Manca, C., and Mora, G. (2001). Non-biomedical health care practices in the State of Morelos, Mexico: Analysis of an emergent phenomenon. *Sociology of Health & Illness, 23*(1), 3–23.

Povinelli, E.A. (1995). Do rocks listen? The cultural politics of apprehending Australian Aboriginal labor. *American Anthropologist, 97*(3), 505–518.

Prufer, K.M. (2006). Animatism. In J.H. Birx, ed., *Encyclopedia of anthropology* (p. 79). Thousand Oaks, CA: Sage.

Reece, G.J. (2010). Shamanism. In J.H. Birx, ed., *21st century anthropology: A reference handbook* (pp. 1–10). Los Angeles, CA: Sage.

Rountree, K. (2012). Neo-paganism, animism, and kinship with nature. *Journal of Contemporary Religion, 27*(2), 305–320.

Saladin d'Anglure, B. (1996). Shamanism. In A. Barnard and J. Spencer, eds., *Encyclopedia of social and cultural anthropology* (pp. 504–508). London: Routledge.

Schilling, C. (1993). *The body and social theory.* London: Sage.

Trotter, R.T., and Chavira, J.A. (1997). *Curanderismo: Mexican American folk healing.* Athens: University of Georgia Press.

Tylor, E.B. (1913). *Primitive culture: Researches into the development of mythology, philosophy, religion, language, art, and custom.* London: Murray. (Originally published in 1871.)

Vaneigem, R. (2012). *The revolution of everyday life.* Oakland, CA: PM Press. (Originally published in 1967.)

Viesca, C. (1997). *Ticiotl: Conceptos médicos de los antiquos mexicanos.* Monografías de Historia y Filosofía de la Medicina, Núm. 2, Mexico City: Universidad Nacional Autónoma de México.

Vitebsky, P. (2003). From cosmology to environmentalism: Shamanism as local knowledge in a global setting. In G. Harvey, ed., *Shamanism: A reader* (pp. 276–298). London: Routledge.

Viveiros de Castro, E. (1998). Cosmological deixis and Amerindian perspectivism. *Journal of the Royal Anthropological Institute, 4*(3), 469–488.

Von Stuckrad, K. (2002). Re-enchanting nature: Modern Western shamanism and nineteenth-century thought. *Journal of the American Academy of Religion, 70*(4), 771–799.

Von Stuckrad, K. (2003). *Schamanismus und Esoterik: Kultur- und wissenschaftsgeschichtliche Betrachtungen*. Leuven, Belgium: Peeters.

Wallis, R.J. (2003). *Shamans/neo-shamans: Ecstasy, alternative archaeologies and contemporary pagans*. London: Routledge.

Wallis, R.J. (2009). Re-enchanting rock art landscapes: Animic ontologies, nonhuman agency and rhizomic personhood. *Time & Mind: The Journal of Archaeology, Consciousness and Culture, 2*(1), 47–69.

Whyte, S.R. (2009). Health identities and subjectivities. *Medical Anthropology Quarterly, 23*(1), 6–15.

Wörrle, B. (2002). *Heiler, Rituale und Patienten: Schamanismus in den Anden Ecuadors*. Berlin: Reimer.

Part II
TRANSFORMATIONS IN HEALTHCARE POLICY—
Politics and ethics

3   Selling global HPV

Pharmaceutical marketing and healthcare policymaking in the case of human papillomavirus vaccination in Austria and Japan

Bernhard Hadolt and Monika Gritsch

Introduction

Infections with human papillomaviruses (HPV) and associated social practices are noteworthy, even remarkable, in several regards. Here are some of them: With an infection rate of up to 80% of the world's population, virtually 'all of us'—meaning sexually active humans—have it, or have already had it, or will have it perhaps again. There is not one single HPV strain, but more than 100 different genotypes and even more are still being discovered. About 30 of them affect anogenital tissues and are primarily transmitted by sexual contact (if not necessarily sexual intercourse), making HPV the proximate cause for the most common sexually transmitted infections. Most of these infections are transient and go unnoticed. When persistent, HPV may induce benign genital warts (low-risk HPVs, predominantly strains 6 and 11) and, above all, cervical and other anogenital and oropharyngeal cancers (in particular associated with the high-risk strains 16 and 18). Thus it appears that HPVs profoundly redefine these cancers, particularly cervical cancer, as infectious, sexually transmitted diseases.

Yet, the link between HPVs and the diseases concerned is far from being deterministic. Having been exposed to HPV, someone may or may not be infected and subsequently may or may not develop warts or cancers. The causal connection between exposure, infection, and resulting diseases has been established by statistical probability. According to the Deutsches Krebsforschungszentrum (German Centre for Cancer Research), 'less than one in 100 women infected with one of the high risk types will develop a cervical carcinoma on an average of fifteen years after the initial infection' (DKFZ, 2009).

However, the pharmaceutical industry was able to provide good news: In 2006, Merck & Co. (in Europe represented by Sanofi Pasteur MSD) introduced Gardasil, an HPV vaccine against strains 6, 11, 16, and 18; one year later GlaxoSmithKline (GSK) launched Cervarix, a bivalent serum against strains 16 and 18. Since these viruses are supposedly transmitted during first sexual contact, both vaccines predominantly targeted girls and young women prior to their first sexual experiences.[1]

In subsequent years, GSK and Merck & Co. introduced their vaccines in more and more national healthcare systems, starting with rich industrialized countries in Europe, North America, Australia, and Japan. Today, millions of girls and young women around the world are vaccinated. However, it is still unknown how long protection against HPV infection lasts (ECDC, 2012). Thus, even those who are vaccinated may not feel safe.

Instead, it is quite likely that they will be infected at least once in the course of their sexually active lives with one of the other HPV types that are not targeted by the vaccines. And it is all but certain that these women will transmit one of the potentially malign viruses to their sexual partners.

In 2006/2007 the general public as well as health policymakers, physicians, and social scientists not only learned about HPV-induced diseases and the new vaccines for the first time, but also about HPV itself: a specifically configured entity that did not exist in the public domain until then— despite the fact that according to biological and medical experts it is an age-old virus that has been afflicting mankind since its dawn. Countries subsequently responded quite differently to this 'new' agent and to the availability of HPV vaccines both in terms of public debates and health policymaking.

In this contribution, we look at how HPV vaccination has become (or has not become) part of public health programmes from a comparative perspective, using the cases of Austria and Japan.[2] Based on analysis of interviews with actors in the field, media accounts, and websites, as part of ongoing ethnographic studies in both countries, we focus particularly on interrelations between public debates and policymaking involving HPV vaccinations, on the one hand, and marketing strategies of the pharmaceutical industry, on the other.

Public health policies, not only in the case of HPV vaccination, involve claims of care. While physicians working in clinical practice and national politicians usually limit their arguments about HPV to a local, national level, the pharmaceutical industry represents itself as responsible and competent 'for battling disease and promoting wellness on a global scale', as Merck &

---

1   Meanwhile the age limit for women has been abrogated; boys and young men may be vaccinated up to age 26 (Gritsch, 2012, p. 73).

2   We wish to thank all our informants for their willingness to share their knowledge and viewpoints with us. Bernhard Hadolt also thanks Hagiwara Takuya and Shimoda Motomu for their support with data collection in Japan when he stayed as a visiting professor at the Institute for Research in Humanities, Kyoto University, in 2011.

Co. claims.[3] For pharmaceutical companies, introducing a drug in a new market requires adjusting organizational tasks to local conditions, such as ensuring the availability of the drug, setting up pathways for its distribution, and making decisions about pricing. In addition, it also entails a 'downscaling' of the globally constructed meanings of the drug to the local level, in other words, framing the need for a drug in medical terms, envisioning its benefits, defining target groups, etc., yet with close reference to and as part of claims of global care.

In order to achieve the goal of creating and pushing a global demand for their vaccines, pharmaceutical companies themselves act globally and, to a remarkable degree, in accordance with one another. Kalman Applbaum (2006), in discussing the introduction of new antidepressants to the Japanese health market, identifies a key element in these concerted strategies. Unlike some 15 years ago, pharmaceutical products themselves are today no longer altered to best suit their regional environment: 'Instead, firms are working strategically and in some regards cooperatively to alter the total environment in which these drugs are or may be used', thus creating a 'new paradigm in pharmaceutical marketing: the *global drug-marketing platform*''' (Applbaum, 2006, pp. 86–87, emphasis added).

We argue that in the case of HPV vaccination, Austria and Japan are engaged with this global drug-marketing platform through which transnational pharmaceutical corporations seek to market their vaccines with high revenues. By comparing these two countries as they have been engaged with HPV vaccination up until the time of writing in 2013, we seek to shed light on how global marketing and the flow of commodities and services engage different localities in specific configurations and vice versa.

Global HPV

HPV and its associated diseases are global phenomena, which have created equally large global markets for the pharmaceutical companies. In 2008, only two years after the launch of Merck's Gardasil, the vaccine was sold for US$1.4 billion (Merck & Co., 2009), albeit almost exclusively in the rich countries of the North and West. It was only later that GSK and Merck & Co. started to provide their products on a larger scale in less developed areas, transforming those regions into so-called emerging markets. In these

3   'About us', Merck website, http://www.merck.com/about/our-values/home.html [last accessed: 15 September 2013].

countries the burden of disease with regard to cervical cancer is generally much higher, as access to effective measures for early-stage diagnosis, in particular Pap smear screening and treatment, is often virtually inexistent. Of the approximately 275,000 women who die from cervical cancer every year, 88% (242,000 women) live in the developing world (Sichero and Villa, 2013, p. 84). It is often argued in national HPV debates that cervical carcinoma is the second-leading cause of all cancer-related female deaths. Considering the numbers above, this argument only holds if women worldwide are taken into account. In industrialized countries it does not come second: in the UK, death from cervical cancer ranks seventeenth,[4] in Austria twelfth, and in Japan eleventh (Piso, 2010; Hamashima et al., 2010).

In the wealthy, industrialized world, the vaccines were marketed rather strenuously as soon as they were allowed to enter the market, despite the fact that cervical cancer, in epidemiological terms, is not a major health problem in these countries. For the same reason, there has been serious opposition to the preventative vaccination of healthy (uninfected) young girls. Both these debates and the national policies for the implementation of HPV vaccination demonstrate significant national differences that can be contributed to a variety of associated sociocultural and historical factors. For example, in the discussion in Germany, the medicalization of healthy girls at a young age, the problematization of adolescent sexual behaviour, the exploitation of mothers' sense of responsibility for their daughters' healthy futures, and the supposed profiteering of the pharmaceutical industry were main issues (Sabisch, 2009; Kolip and Schach, 2010). In the UK, the introduction of the HPV vaccination was profoundly influenced by two controversies concerning infant organ transplantation in the 1990s and the measles, mumps, and rubella (MMR) vaccine in 1998. Both 'influenced the public's trust in vaccination programmes, however, parental opposition to the HPV vaccine was based on concerns about the vaccine's long-term safety and questions about whether or not one could trust public health officials' (Stöckl, 2010, p. 259). Not least, in many countries including Germany and the United States, questions were also raised concerning vaccine safety (Sabisch, 2009; Casper and Carpenter, 2008).

GSK, Merck & Co., and Sanofi Pasteur MSD acted and reacted deliberately in regard to the diversities of regional health markets, as we demonstrate below for Austria and Japan. On a global scale their discursive strategies

4   'Cervical cancer mortality statistics', Cancer Research UK website, http://www.cancer-researchuk.org/cancer-info/cancerstats/types/cervix/mortality/uk-cervical-cancer-mortality-statistics#world [last accessed: 15 September 2013].

for introducing their upscale products show some recurring elements: an emphasis on altruistic motives in the public interest, the staging and exploitation of the fear of catching a contagious disease and developing cancer respectively (Gritsch, 2012, p. 93), and the claim to possess what Jordan (1997) calls 'authoritative knowledge'. By that she means 'the knowledge that participants agree counts in a particular situation, that *they* see as consequential, on the basis of which *they* make decisions and provide justifications for courses of action' (Jordan, 1997, p. 58; emphasis in original).

The discursive production of fear associated with HPV deserves particular attention, as it constitutes a main method in the marketing strategies of the pharmaceutical industry in order to alter the 'total sales environment' and hence develop key markets. This can be understood as being part of what medical sociologists Williams and colleagues (2011), conceptualizing the ongoing processes of the pharmaceuticalization of societies, refer to as 'disease mongering' and 'selling sickness'. They define this as:

> a process in which the social construction of illness is being replaced by the 'corporate construction of disease'. [...] This involves: (i) turning ordinary ailments into medical problems; (ii) seeing mild symptoms as serious; (iii) treating personal problems as medical; (iv) seeing risks as diseases; and (v) framing prevalence estimates to maximize potential markets. (Williams et al., 2011, p. 713)

Disease mongering as a corporate construction of HPV-related suffering is closely connected to the production of HPV itself as a killer of women, a dangerous, contagious agent causing sickness, cancer, and death. This entity was not only new to the public, but via its connection to cervical cancer it also became highly gendered, thus creating a huge target group and conceptualizing women—once again—as one category: cervical cancer requires having a uterus. Consequently, as the U.S. Centers for Disease Control and Prevention puts it, '[a]ll women are at risk for cervical cancer',[5] and girls, young women, and mothers all around the world thus need to be not only informed, but educated. For several years only Austria, Australia, and the United States recommended HPV vaccination for both girls and boys (Kunze and Böhm, 2010, p. 658), but still emphasizing women as the primary concern. Only recently have boys and men received more attention as possible target groups for vaccination—not only as carriers of HPVs and

---

5   Centers for Disease Control and Prevention, U.S. Department of Health and Human Services, http://www.cdc.gov/cancer/cervical/pdf/cervical_facts.pdf [last accessed: 15 September 2013]

sufferers from genital warts, but also as possible victims of HPV-related cancers (Giuliano et al., 2011; Newman et al., 2013).

HPV in Austria

Austria was the first European country that recommended the vaccines despite having an effective cervical cancer prevention programme already in place since the late 1960s. The programme consists of opportunistic, cost-free, Pap smear screening, recommended annually for all women aged 20 or older. Haidinger and colleagues (2008, p. 222) report: 'In 2005, 95.7% of all women aged 20–69 years knew about Pap smear screening (1995: 94.0%), and 88.0% were screened at least once (1995: 76.2%). 52.6% of all women can be classified as having been screened optimally.' Cancer incidence and mortality have constantly decreased since the implementation of the programme. At the time of writing, every year about 380 Austrian women are diagnosed with cervical carcinoma and about 140 die from it (Statistik Austria, 2011a, 2011b).

Nevertheless, when Gardasil and Cervarix were introduced in 2006 and 2007 respectively, their promotion as a 'vaccine against cervical cancer' worked well, and Austrian media, physicians, and health politicians were all in favour of widespread vaccination coverage. Educational work and aware-ness campaigns funded in part by the pharmaceutical industry amplified consent in the public sphere, too. 'The acceptance for our vaccine in Austria was spectacular!', recalled a pharmaceutical marketing manager to whom we talked about the market developments at that point. He continued: 'The sales figures per capita were higher than in any other country'.

But soon the debates and attitudes changed, leading Austrian HPV policy down a very different path. By early 2008, when the HPV debate in Germany was at its peak (Sabisch, 2009), in Austria the topic had already vanished from newspapers, talk shows, and the public interest in general (Gritsch, 2012). As of October 2013, the vaccination rate in Austria is still lower than 5%, compared to up to 90% of girls and young women in Great Britain, Australia, and Canada; and up to 60% in Germany, France, and Belgium (Hörandl, 2010).

As to the historical processes that led to this situation, the stakeholders in the field seem to share a consistent view, summarized by one of our informants, who is an expert in social medicine at the Medical University of Vienna, as an 'unfortunate mix of misinformation', involving the discur-sive entanglement of the vaccination and the death of a nineteen-year-old

Austrian woman in October 2007. Despite an autopsy report that could not substantiate a causal relation to the dose administered, there was a short but violent flare-up of the topic in Austrian media, which led to considerable anxiety about the vaccine, not only in the public, but also among many gynaecologists. In addition, in early 2008 the then Austrian health minister Andrea Kdolsky decided not to subsidize HPV vaccination (by incorporating it into the national vaccination programme) due to its extraordinary high price (see also Stöckl, 2010). 'Because of all these factors', the medical expert continued, 'HPV vaccination is dead and virtually non-existent in our country'. Similarly, a representative of the pharmaceutical industry described the HPV vaccine as a 'burnt-out' topic in Austria.

Arguments employed by stakeholders in the field to interpret this Austrian development vary, depending on individual positioning for or against vaccination. It seems that on a pragmatic level, the vaccine manufacturers' original price led to a stand-off between industry and politics: the Ministry of Health did not accept the costs to its budget; the Austrian branch offices of the pharmaceutical companies showed an unwillingness to negotiate. Subsequently, not least due to the commissions required by their parent companies, they withdrew from the Austrian market. A spokesperson of the medical profession told us: 'On the one hand patients mostly are not able to afford these prices,[6] and on the other there are the huge corporations. The local firms are not allowed to do what they want, and the parent companies don't care about whether a handful of Austrians get vaccinated or not'. Consequently, most of the industry's awareness-raising campaigns concerning HPV vaccination were almost completely halted, which led to a considerable lack of knowledge about HPVs not only in the public sphere but also in the medical domain.

In 2011, the issue of HPV vaccination re-entered the political stage: GSK and Sanofi Pasteur MSD established a joint HPV working group with the dual goal of raising awareness among Austrian healthcare policy stakeholders and disseminating new information. A GSK spokesperson explained this step to us in the following way: 'Considering the Austrian situation right now, it does not make sense to act solitarily. It is more reasonable to form one interlocutor who also gets acknowledged as a partner by public authorities.'

Additionally, the companies reduced the high prices of their vaccines to a more moderate level and resumed negotiations with the Austrian Ministry of Health for subsidizing vaccination within the national vaccination

6   The original price for a complete immunization with either vaccine was €624 (€208 per dose).

programme. Consequently, as of 2012 mentions of the vaccination and the virus began to reappear on a sporadic but a regular basis in the Austrian media and medical journals. Finally, in August 2013 Health Minister Alois Stöger declared that, starting in February 2014, vaccination would be state funded for children aged nine as part of a school-based HPV vaccination programme.

What is remarkable here is the inclusion of boys in the vaccination programme alongside girls. As the first European country to subsidize HPV vaccination for boys, Austria is resuming its leading role in making HPV a relevant issue for both women and men, as it had done when it recommended HPV vaccination for both girls and boys in 2006. This Austrian policy decision lines up with a general change in discourse. While boys were mainly seen affected as transmitters of HPVs until recently, they are now becoming increasingly perceived as potential sufferers from HPV-related cancers.

HPV in Japan

GSK's Cervarix was first to launch in Japan in December 2009, and Merck & Co. followed with Gardasil in September 2011. Compared to the launches of HPV vaccines in other parts of the world, this was a rather late development. This 'vaccine gap' (Saitoh and Okabe, 2012) of about three years seems to have been due to the Japanese drug-approval procedure that requires pharmaceutical corporations to submit additional clinical trials done in Japan because of the supposed physiological specificities of Japanese people (see also Applbaum, 2006). However, according to a GSK sales manager, this 'vaccine gap' of about three or four years, which, compared to other pharmaceutical fields, was rather short, had the advantage that Japan's branch of GSK already had knowledge about 'what is going on globally' and could adjust their marketing strategies accordingly.

As several Japanese gynaecologists have complained in interviews, gynaecological check-up rates in Japan are rather low, particularly the rate of Pap smear test as a preventive measure against cervical cancer, with an estimated number of 15,000 women developing cervical cancer per year, and 3500 women dying from it. Women in their 30s and 40s in particular do not have gynaecological check-ups, since, according to interviewed gynaecologists, they conceive of cancer and other gynaecological problems as older women's problems. In Japan, the Pap smear rate now is about 40%, but only a couple of years ago was around 20%; compare this, for example, to the rate in the United States of about 85% (OECD, 2013).

This fact is significant in at least two regards: First, young women in Japan neither knew nor cared much about cervical cancer and the risk of developing the disease, at least until Cervarix entered the scene. Second, the low rates of Pap smear tests enforced the argument that HPV vaccination was urgently needed in order to save women from dying of cervical cancer. Both points were explicitly voiced as urgent rationales for vaccination by practically all stakeholders in the policymaking process, and especially by gynaecologists.

When GSK launched Cervarix in Japan, the company had to 'start from scratch' and 'dig into the market', as the GSK sales manager put it. Besides getting the vaccine approved GSK took major efforts to 'raise awareness' about both cervical cancer and the fact that HPV vaccination can prevent cervical cancer. According to the GSK sales manager they had to educate all people involved: mothers, girls, young women, media people, local and national policymakers, and not least doctors. They did so using multiple strategies.

The key message geared towards the public at the time of the vaccine's launch in 2009 was the same as in other countries and comprised three dimensions: every woman has a risk of developing cervical cancer, the cause of cervical cancer is HPV, and HPV vaccination can prevent it and consequently save lives. GSK spread this message through manifold channels, including newspaper articles, TV advertisements, radio features, and the organization of public discussions as part of a large-scale, direct-to-consumer advertising campaign. The company collaborated with self-help groups, advocacy groups (such as the Japan Cancer Association), and doctor's associations (such as the Japan Gynaecology Association and the Japan Society of Gynaecologists and Oncology).

According to the GSK sales manager, within a few years awareness about cervical cancer and HPV vaccination rose from a very low level up to 90% of Japanese women due to such activities. In 2011 GSK shifted its key message to a 'higher level', as the sales manager put it, also stressing the importance of Pap smear testing. He explained:

> [W]e are a pharmaceutical company selling a vaccine but we have to deliver the message about screening as well. [...] We have to say: The vaccine is not perfect and cervical cancer is only perfectly prevented both by screening and the vaccine. So we shift to the other message as well and [put] more weight on the screening because we are quite afraid that

some people will misunderstand: 'Oh, I got the vaccine and I never will get cervical cancer'. And 10 years later she has no Pap smear, then gets cancer. It's possible, so there is quite a worst [case] scenario for us as well.

The sales manager repeatedly stressed the importance of safety issues for GSK's marketing strategies as: 'Japanese are very, very, very, sensitive about safety'. In particular, he thought that rather than weighing benefits against risk, many Japanese people would not consider vaccination at all if concerns about major side effects of the vaccine were raised.

As the prime message of GSK's awareness-raising activities was focused on the protection of women from cervical cancer, the fact that other HPV-related cancers might be a health problem too hardly surfaced in the debate. This was even more the case with the notion that men also might benefit from vaccination and hence boys should be vaccinated alongside girls. The sales manager justified GSK's decision to not submit its vaccine for approval for boys as well by referring to limited public health funds and women being the primary beneficiaries of the vaccine. In their awareness-rising activities, GSK furthermore aimed to omit, as much as possible, the fact that HPVs are transmitted via sexual contact, because they feared that the issue would be misconstrued as encouraging sex among girls at a younger age. Female promiscuity had already become an issue in the public HPV debate in the United Kingdom, among other places (see Hilton et al., 2010; Stöckl, 2010).

The ultimate goal, according to the sales manager, was to make HPV vaccination an ordinary thing to do: 'Japanese people tend to follow everybody else: When everyone does it, I do. [...] So when everyone starts [doing] it, the rest of the population starts to follow'. Alongside the consideration of safety issues, the elision of HPV as being sexually transmitted was considered a key aspect in developing, in the words of the sales manager, 'our own way' of promoting HPV vaccination in Japan.

Expert knowledge about cervical cancer and HPV vaccination was also spread to doctors, in particular gynaecologists, paediatricians, and internists. GSK trained doctors, organized seminars, and contributed to major conferences for the Japan Association of Obstetricians and Gynaecologists and the Japan Society of Gynaecologic Oncology where topics associated with cervical cancer and HPV vaccination were discussed. The company also collaborated with researchers at high-ranking Japanese universities, such as Osaka University, to gather epidemiological data on the prevalence of HPV infection and the long-term effectiveness of HPV vaccination in Japan. Additionally, GSK provided health policymakers and civil servants with cervical cancer-related information, lobbied for a fast approval of its vaccine, and advocated that HPV vaccination be financed with public funds.

On the whole, GSK was indeed successful in regulating the flow of information about cervical cancer and HPV vaccination in Japan by the time Merck & Co. entered the market with Gardasil in 2011. Most interviewed stakeholders referred to informational materials that had been distributed by GSK when asked about the source of their knowledge. Furthermore, consensus about the effectiveness and safety of Cervarix among stakeholders was high at that time. Health officials from one major city reported that all of Japan's major cities planned to petition the national government to make HPV vaccination mandatory for girls.

As early as spring and summer 2010, several local governments throughout Japan started to cover all or part of the costs of approximately ¥50,000 (about €400) for immunization with Cervarix (Fujiwara et al., 2011; Hayashi et al., 2012). By the end of 2010, the national government announced the establishment of an HPV vaccination fund; in February 2011 this fund in cooperation with local governments began fully subsidizing the vaccine for girls aged twelve to sixteen. According to GSK, in summer 2011 the average vaccination rate already was about 50% for this age cohort. This interim nationwide programme was made permanent when in April 2013 HPV vaccination became included in the national immunization programme following a revision of the Japanese Preventive Vaccination Act.

However, only a few months later, in June 2013, the Ministry of Health, Labour, and Welfare withdrew its recommendation for HPV vaccination, following reports of several cases of supposed significant side effects including severe pain, convulsions, and numbness. Two medical expert groups were set up by the ministry to examine these cases. At the time of writing, findings of such investigations have not yet been made public and the Japanese HPV-vaccination policy continues to be marked by a situation in which the vaccine is still available free of charge, yet without the governmental recommendation for its use. Thus, a development that looked favourable to pharmaceutical interests has taken quite a sudden turn of events.

Concluding remarks

A new paradigm of pharmaceutical marketing, the global drug-marketing platform (Applbaum, 2006), alters 'total sales environments' to make them fit for pharmaceutical products. Such environments include not only policy and economic factors, but also people's ideas and behaviours, which are modified by persuading them that they are not well and are in need of drugs to get well again. Concerning preventive vaccines, this entails a shift from present to future problems, to diseases that are prognosticated instead of diagnosed. Consequently, the making of 'being at risk' is most crucial here, since the industry's success requires people to become aware that they face possible disease and mortal danger.

In the case of the rapid implementation of HPV vaccination into health-care services in the industrialized world, this marketing of risk has involved a number of discursive elements. These include the highly gendered 'disease mongering' (Williams et al., 2011) of cervical cancer as a major killer of women, the redefinition of cervical cancer as being caused by HPV, and the assertion that virtually 'all of us' carry the virus. The discursive association of the fear-laden ideas of cancer, virus, contagion, and sexual transmissibility sustained the marketing message about the HPV vaccine being a 'vaccine against cancer', rather than a vaccine against a virus, or against specific strains of HPV. On the whole, HPV vaccination was framed predominantly in medical terms.

In both Austria and Japan, this discursive configuration constituted the basis on which national debates were shaped and pharmaceutical industry marketing strategies were built: enrolling medical associations and patient support groups for awareness-raising campaigns, providing authoritative knowledge to politicians via lobbying, and using a rhetoric of altruistic motives and public interest with the media. Together these constitute an encompassing strategy of change, exemplifying what a global drug-marketing platform looks like in the case of HPV vaccines. At first glance, the Austrian situation seemed early on to be a case of the potential failure of the pharmaceutical marketing strategies described. At the local level, this might have been the case, notwithstanding the fact that Austria recently has joined other industrialized countries in subsidizing HPV vaccination. But put in a global context it proves otherwise: it is economically all too logical that globally active companies withdraw a product from a rather small, unviable market such as Austria when marketing strategies are not successful.

The cases of Austria and Japan also show that while the broad lines of the above discursive configuration were the same, they were also shaped by distinctive local conditions. In Austria, as in other countries such as Germany and the United Kingdom, a counterdiscourse surfaced within a short time after the public debate started that was critical of HPV vaccinations. This counterdiscourse highlighted possible deficiencies of the vaccine, including adverse side effects, and its low benefits in a situation where an effective screening programme was already long in place. In a cost-benefit calculation, the risk of developing cancer was weighed against the risk of side effects, and the public costs for HPV vaccination weighed against the benefits of investing in other health areas. In addition, the issue of boys as possible beneficiaries of the vaccine was part of the discussion right from the beginning.

In Japan, the situation was almost reversed: until recently, the pharmaceutical companies, particularly GSK, dominated the dissemination of HPV-related information and both the risk of severe side effects and the fact that HPVs are sexually transmitted were carefully avoided. The issue of boys as a target group for vaccination was set aside in the drug-approval procedure, in the public debate, as well as in the policymaking process. In order to find a 'Japanese way' of promoting HPV vaccination, GSK also prioritized making it an ordinary thing to do, so that most people would follow the vaccination recommendations once set in motion. When major safety concerns finally did emerge, they radically marginalized the talk about possible benefits of the vaccination and state authorities had to withdraw their recommendation for vaccination.

The cases of Austria and Japan highlight that the marketing of drugs has to be understood as a process that may include sharp turns, as demonstrated in Austria by the policy shift towards state-subsidized HPV vaccination, and in Japan by the shift away from state support of the vaccine. These idiographic situations and processes show that the global drug-marketing platform works in a multidirectional fashion rather than as a one-way street. While local environments are indeed altered in order to become receptive to pharmaceutical products, this to some extent also applies to the global marketing programme and products. By way of actively adjusting their marketing strategies to local needs and circumstances, products are also 'adjusted': some of their properties become highlighted and others downplayed. By carefully modifying the meaning of a pharmaceutical product, a kind of 'contact zone' is constituted between the product, local discourses, and medical practices that may make it appropriate for implementation. It is along this global/local contact zone that authoritative knowledges, fears of a disease-infested future, and rhetorics of (global) care and promised cures are played out—together giving form to new disease entities, risky selves, and new markets.

References

Applbaum, K. (2006). Educating for global mental health: The adoption of SSRIs in Japan. In A. Petryna, A. Lakoff, and A. Kleinman, eds., *Global pharmaceuticals: Ethics, markets, practices* (pp. 85–110). Durham: Duke University Press.

Casper, M.J., and Carpenter, L.M. (2008). Sex, drugs, and politics: The HPV vaccine for cervical cancer. *Sociology of Health & Illness, 30*(6), 886–899.

DKFZ (2009). HPV als Krebsrisiko: Humane Papillomaviren als Krebsauslöser: Sind Warzenviren wirklich so gefährlich? Deutsches Krebsforschungszentrum. Retrieved from http://www.krebsinformationsdienst.de/vorbeugung/risiken/hpv.php.

ECDC (2012). *Introduction of HPV vaccines in European Union countries: An update.* Stockholm: European Centre for Disease Prevention and Control.

Fujiwara, H., Yoshinari, T., and Shiiya, K. (2011). Free school-based vaccination with HPV vaccine in a Japanese city. *Vaccine, 29*, 6441–6442.

Giuliano, A.R., Palefsky, J.M., and Goldstone, S. (2011). Efficacy of quadrivalent HPV vaccine against HPV infection and disease in males. *New England Journal of Medicine, 364*(5), 401–411.

Gritsch, M. (2012). *HPV–eine widersprüchliche Karriere: Zur Situation der HPV-Impfung in Österreich.* Unpublished master's thesis. University of Vienna, Vienna, Austria.

Haidinger, G., Waldhoer, T., and Vutuc, C. (2008). Self-reported pap smear screening in Austria. *Wiener Medizinische Wochenschrift, 158*(7–8), 222–226.

Hamashima, C., et al. (2010). The Japanese guideline for cervical cancer screening. *Japanese Journal of Clinical Oncology, 40*(6), 485–502.

Hayashi, Y., Shimizu, Y., Netsu, S., Hanley, S. J., and Konno, R. (2012). High HPV vaccination uptake rates for adolescent girls after regional governmental funding in Shiki City, Japan. *Vaccine, 30*, 5547–5550.

Hilton, S., Hunt, K., Langan, M., Bedford, H., and Petticrew, M. (2010). Newsprint media representations of the introduction of the HPV vaccination programme for cervical cancer prevention in the UK (2005–2008). *Social Science & Medicine, 70*(6), 942–950.

Hörandl, F. (2010). *HPV-Infektionen: Effektiver Schutz durch primäre Prävention.* Retrieved from http://haematologie-onkologie.universimed.com/artikel/hpv-infektionen-effektiver-schutz-durch-prim%C3%A4re-pr%C3%A4vention.

Jordan, B. (1997). Authoritative knowledge and its construction. In R.E. Davis-Floyd and C.F. Sargent, eds., *Childbirth and authoritative knowledge: Cross-cultural perspectives* (pp. 55–79). Berkeley: University of California Press.

Kolip, P., and Schach, C. (2010). Impfung gegen Krebs?: HPV-Impfung und die Gesundheit von Mädchen und jungen Frauen. In P. Kolip and J. Lademann, eds., *Frauenblicke auf das Gesundheitssystem: Frauengerechte Gesundheitsversorgung zwischen Marketing und Ignoranz* (pp. 23–38). Weinheim: Juventa Verlag.

Kunze, U. and Böhm, G. (2010). Public health analyse—Humane Papillomviren Daten und Fakten für Österreich. *Wiener Klinische Wochenschrift, 122*(23), 655–659.

Merck & Co. (2009). *Annual report 2008 on form 10-K.* Retrieved from http://www.merck.com/investors/financials/annual-reports/home.html.

Newman, P.A., Logie, C.H., Doukas, N., and Asakura, K. (2013). HPV vaccine acceptability among men: A systematic review and meta-analysis. *Sexually Transmitted Infections, 89*, 568–574. doi:10.1136/sextrans-2012-050980.

OECD (2013). Screening, survival and mortality for cervical cancer. In *Health at a Glance 2013: OECD Indicators* (pp. 124–125). Paris: Organisation for Economic Co-operation and Development. doi:10.1787/health_glance-2013-51-en.

Petryna, A., and Kleinman, A. (2006). The pharmaceutical nexus. In A. Petryna, A. Lakoff, and A. Kleinman, eds., *Global pharmaceuticals: Ethics, markets, practices* (pp. 1–32). Durham: Duke University Press.

Piso, B. (2010). Angst und Hoffnung: Die Impfung gegen Krebs. In C. Wild and B. Piso, eds., *Zahlenspiele in der Medizin: Eine kritische Analyse* (pp. 79–90). Vienna: Orac.

Sabisch, K. (2009). Hoffnungslos durchseucht: Zur diskursiven Infektiosität des Humanen Papilloma Virus in den deutschen Medien, 2006–2009. *GENDER: Zeitschrift für Geschlecht, Kultur und Gesellschaft, 1*(1), 107–124.

Saitoh, A., and Okabe, N. (2012). Current issues with the immunization program in Japan: Can we fill the 'vaccine gap'? *Vaccine, 30,* 4752–4756.

Sichero, L., and Villa, L.L. (2013). HPV and cervical cancer. In M.K. Shetty, ed., *Breast and gynecological cancers: An integrated approach for screening and early diagnosis in developing countries* (pp. 83–98). New York: Springer.

Statistik Austria (2011a). *Gebärmutterhals (C53)–Krebsinzidenz (Neuerkrankungen pro Jahr), Österreich ab 1983.* Retreived from https://www.statistik.at/web_de/ statistiken/gesundheit/ krebserkrankungen/gebaermutterhals/index.html.

Statistik Austria (2011b). *Gebärmutterhals (C53)–Krebsmortalität (Sterbefälle pro Jahr), Österreich ab 1983.* Retrieved from https://www.statistik.at/web_de/ gesundheit/ krebserkrankungen/gebaermutterhals/index.html.

Stöckl, A. (2010). Public discourses and policymaking: The HPV vaccination from the European perspective. In K. Wailoo, J. Livingston, S. Epstein, and R. Aronowitz, eds., *Three shots at prevention: The HPV vaccine and the politics of medicine's simple solutions* (pp. 254–269). Baltimore, MD: Johns Hopkins University Press.

Williams, S.J., Martin, P., and Gae, J. (2011). The pharmaceuticalisation of society? A framework for analysis. *Sociology of Health & Illness, 33*(5), 710–725.

4   The birth of disabled people as 'ambiguous citizens'

Biopolitics, the ethical regime of the impaired body, and the ironies of identity politics in Thailand

Prachatip Kata

Introduction

I remember well the day I first met Sak, a blind man in his 50s who earns a living as a singer in the streets of Bangkok. Our meeting took place at a market in a large government agency compound, which houses many government offices. As Sak sang, he periodically bent his head down, as if shy. He was holding a microphone in his right hand and a small wooden donation box in his left; on his back he was carrying a shabby-looking loudspeaker. At the end of Sak's working day, I interviewed him and Thida, his wife.

'Coming out to sing like this, are you not scared of being arrested by the social welfare officers or the city police officers?' I asked Sak, posing a question to which I had been curious to know the answer. He responded, 'I have never been arrested, but many of my friends have. Those who are arrested and thrown in a "public welfare shelter" are mostly accused of being "homeless beggars", an illegal activity. If no relatives bail such people out, they may be stuck in a shelter for a long time. My friends tell me that it is very scary there.' Sak paused, as if thinking of something. 'At the shelter the fence is very high, and buildings separate the men from the women. When it is bedtime, the lights are switched off, and the attendants at the shelter drag their batons along the floor while patrolling and counting those staying there. They always keep their ears open, to hear if anyone dares to answer back, and if someone does, that person is beaten.'

He then told me that a few years before, the governor of Bangkok had launched a policy to "sweep up" the homeless people and the foreign beggars in Bangkok. However, blind singers found walking on pedestrian walkways or stationed on pedestrian bridges were also arrested by the officers. Sometimes, when the officers came to arrest groups of foreign beggars at the apartment blocks where the blind singers also lived, the blind singers were also arrested. Sak referred to this as the 'arresting era'.

I planned to interview Sak and his wife again when I returned to meet them the next week. Unfortunately, I was unable to locate Sak and his wife at the market on the following Wednesday, nor any Wednesday after that. I did not know why they changed their location. I coincidentally met them many months later at a Monday market at a university campus. One day, a few months after we had reconnected, Thida revealed the reason why they had not returned to the Wednesday market where I first met them:

> Sak thought you were a social welfare officer or a city police officer in disguise, trying to obtain information or secrets about *wong gan kon taa bot* [the blind people's society], so he was scared of being arrested and sent to a public welfare shelter again. He was arrested once when he was a teenager. I am not sure if the story he tells of the shelter is about his friends or actually his own experiences, that he was violated and suffered a lot.

Sak's suspicion was the result of the biopolitical changes that have taken place during recent years in Thailand; Didier Fassin calls this 'the embodiment of history' (2007) or 'the embodiment of the past' (2008).

This article is based on ethnographic fieldwork that I conducted among blind singers and musicians working on the streets of Bangkok between 2010 and 2011, as well as analysis of documents and interviews with representatives from governmental and nonprofit organizations in Thailand. My research documents a system of ethics that governs how the Thai population deals with people with disabilities, and how this system is related to a transformation in Thai state policies and the country's economic and political context, as well as the discursive power of international organizations and the beliefs held by Theravada Buddhists. Due to this system of ethics, people living with disabilities are treated as political subjects and problematized as moral–political subjects. The Thai state categorizes disabled people in such a way so as to actually facilitate and guarantee their exclusion from society, in a contradictory form of inclusion–exclusion (Agamben, 1998), and in order to maintain a status quo in which good citizens are those with healthy, fully functioning bodies. Perhaps not surprisingly, this biopolitical inclusion–exclusion used by the Thai state—which places disabled people in the same category as homeless people, beggars, and prostitutes, all of whom should be confined to government-run shelters—conforms perfectly with the ideology of karma and the rhetoric of compassion used by Theravada Buddhism. According to this ideology, disabled people should be hidden within the home and wait for assistance, as objects of charity, in the name of humanitarianism and rhetoric of *ve-tha-na* (feeling of pity).

In this politics of life, people with impaired bodies become ambiguous citizens, as they are neither fully fledged citizens who deserve rights and recognition, nor are they noncitizens to whom the state can only provide humanitarian assistance. Moreover, their impaired bodies are viewed as ambiguous also, as they sit somewhere between the definitions of able bodied and disabled bodied, between fully productive, able-bodied citizens and non-productive, disabled citizens. Related to this are certain ironies inherent in the political struggle for humanitarianism among disabled people in Thailand—people who define their citizenship in terms of their legal rights, based on the politics of identity and human rights' discourses.

Part I: The civil body project and biological discourse

During the Thai state's nation-building era (1938–1957), disabled people did not fit into the new political order. The asymmetrical body of a disabled person did not conform within a system of nationalism whose key principle was based on a biological notion of a pure ethnic Thai race, which was thought of as the core of national identity and unity. A disabled body was considered not fit for military service and uncivilized in a civilized, nation-building era. Thus, disabled people were obstacles to the new political order, impeding the liberal-democratic nation in its quest to eliminate all traces of the former monarchical regime.

After the revolution that toppled the monarchy in 1932, the modern Thai state, by then under a new liberal-democratic regime, paid more attention to the biopolitics of the population. This was especially the case during the administrations of Field Marshal Por Pibunsongkhram, who was Thailand's prime minister for two terms, from 1938 to 1944 and again from 1948 to 1957. Under the Pibun regime, the Thai government attempted to cultivate and disseminate a new political, cultural, and ethical standard among its citizens (Suwannathat–Pian, 1995, pp. 102–151). Such sociocultural reforms were intended to transform ideologies and reshape the minds and habits of Thai people (Kawinraweekun, 2003; Puaksom, 2007), and were essentially centred on the bodies of its citizens. Davisakd Puaksom (2007, p. 176) states there were differences between the bodily ideologies of the old monarchy's regime and the new regime of the liberal-democrats. The new regime not only applied medical knowledge in order to maintain a focus on the body itself, but also used disciplinary power to control the minds and behaviours of the population in all aspects of everyday life.

A state decree, Ratthaniyom, which came into effect in 1939, was issued to change certain aspects of everyday life in Thailand—the way people dressed, ate, slept, and worked, not only to promote the country as a civilized nation, but also to cultivate a new ethic of 'Thai-ness' in the minds of the country's citizens (Suwannathat-Pian, 1995, p. 113; Kasetsiri, 2008, pp. 193, 200–201, 212–213). Ratthaniyom no. 10 demanded that Thai citizens divide their 24-hour schedule into three periods: work/normal activities, recreation, and sleeping. It also stipulated that people must not eat more than four meals a day. There was a one-hour break allowed for lunch, and people were to spend at least one hour exercising after work. The law also said people should sleep for six to eight hours a night, and spend their weekends doing activities that were good for both their bodies and minds (Puaksom, 2007, pp. 191–192).

Under the Pibun regime, nationalism was strengthened through the promotion of a 'national identity' and the creation of an imagined community of Thai-ness, both of which were based on a biological discourse in which the supremacy of the Thai race would lead to the destruction of other minority ethnic groups, inside or outside the country (Suwannathat-Pian, 1995, p. 106; Kasetsiri, 2008, pp. 185–186). This trend could also be seen in the art world, in which paintings and sculptures became more realistic and focused on lean, healthy, muscular, and strong bodies that matched the ideology of the nation-building programme (Prakitnonthakarn, 2009). It is clear that during this period, the image of a healthy body became inextricably linked with the identity of a good Thai citizen. According to the Thai nation-building ideals at the time, unemployed and homeless people were a hindrance; the government compared such people to parasites on the human body, as not only useless but also destructive (Puaksom, 2007, p. 193).

Eugenics was a key concept adopted by the government in order to control the quality of the population and to create new and improved future generations. Creating a population strong and healthy enough to become a productive labour force for the state's manufacturing sector was deemed essential to the nation-building process. As a result, all citizens with hereditary or contagious diseases, or with disabilities, became citizens to be controlled, in order to prevent the infecting of new generations. Taking care of these people with diseases or disabilities was characterized as an ongoing burden for the government (Kawinraweekun, 2003, p. 31). According to the new ethical regime regarding the biopolitics of the population in Thailand, disabled people would become 'biological citizens' (Rose and Novas, 2005), with their citizenship linked to a biological discourse within Thai politics.

Social work as a technology of power

Under Pibun and his nation-building programme, not only was medical knowledge used to ensure future generations of capable and productive citizens, but social knowledge was also used to manipulate the bodies of citizens seen as ineffective and unproductive, and, therefore, unable to contribute to building the nation.

The Social Work Programme was developed in the belief that the well-being of the population depended upon social security. The Thai government at that time viewed social workers as a key tool in implementing policies that would take the country into the future, and created a training programme for them (Chotidilok, 1997, p. 451). Social workers were told to focus on and seek out particular target groups that the government considered helpless and therefore problematic (Poshakrishna, 1986, p. 44), namely the poor, the homeless, beggars, and people with disabilities. The rhetoric of compassion emanating from Theravada Buddhism supported the idea that social workers should help disabled people, based on humanitarian goals. One can see that both Buddhism and the Thai government viewed people with impairments as objects of charity.

At that time, the number of homeless people and beggars in Bangkok increased, and this was thought to negatively affect the population in general, obscure the civilized aspect of the nation's culture, and hinder the government's efforts to create a strong, disciplined, and progressive society (Department of Social Welfare, 1990, pp. 102–103). After establishing the Department of Social Welfare in 1940 to assist helpless people, the Thai government enacted the Beggar Control Act in 1941, which stated that beggars in Bangkok, as well as the elderly and disabled—and especially the mentally disabled who begged along roadsides in Bangkok—were not self-reliant and had nobody to look after them, and should therefore be placed in government-run shelters.

Thailand's first government-run shelter was established in compliance with the Beggar Control Act in order to accommodate those arrested by police officers for begging on the streets of Bangkok (Department of Social Welfare, 1981, p. 146). The shelters were essentially asylums into which beggars, the homeless, and the disabled were thrown, along with various other troublemakers and undesirable people. Such people were therefore kept from society, and prevented from causing disorder in it, though they were given the opportunity to learn new and desirable skills, enabling them to return to society as good, well-functioning citizens.

In Agamben's terms (1998, 2005), we can say that the government-run shelters in this era were constructed as 'states of exception'. Inside the shelters, helpless and homeless people remained under the constant surveillance and regulation of the state. These people became 'bare life': subjected to a mixture of biopower by the modern Thai government and the moral doctrines of Theravada Buddhism. Their bodies formed the threshold between the biobody and the politicized body, or which Agamben called 'zones of indistinction'. Their bodies were excluded by means of inclusion, through the power of state mechanisms and the supervision of Thai government officers, or in other words through the use of 'exclusive inclusion'. By placing people with disabilities in these shelters, the modern Thai state was effectively classifying people living with impairments as 'abandoned citizens', just like beggars, prostitutes, and the homeless.

Sak's tales of life inside the shelter and the power that government officers have over those who reside there clearly reflects the bare life experienced by people with disabilities at the hands of the modern Thai government. Life in the shelters underlines the ambiguous status of the disabled population and questions whether the disabled are valued by the country or not. If people with disabilities are not acknowledged as citizens, the government need only provide social welfare based upon moral reasoning. That is, humanitarianism and in the name of *ve-tha-na*. The social work programme employed by the government during the nation-building era can be seen as reinforcing the view that disabled people are objects of charity.

Both the Beggar Control Act—which categorizes people with disabilities as 'helpless'—and the establishment of shelters for those 'confined citizens', resonate perfectly with the karma ideology of Theravada Buddhism. In Buddhist teaching on karma, disability is believed to be an individual tragedy and payback for bad karma accumulated in a previous life (or in previous lives). This belief requires disabled people to pay back their karmic debt as objects of charity, rather than being capable of actively earning merit and escaping their karmic destiny of being disabled (Riewpaiboon and Blume, 2009, p. xx). This view is confirmed by Kulapa Vajanasara's (2005) review of popular literature from the era, which shows that the image of disabled people in Thailand was one of impairment resulting from sins committed in a former life; the disabled were depicted as helpless people who cannot do anything without the help of others, and as passive objects of charitable action. According to karmic ideology, people with disabilities should be hidden within the home as a family stigma, and should passively wait for assistance. There is no doubt that this Theravada Buddhist idea of disabled people as hidden objects is mirrored in Thai state ideology, in which disabled people should be confined citizens.

Disabled people as a human resource

Between 1970 and 1980, the Thai state was greatly concerned by the increasing number of people with disabilities. Disability was considered to be an outcome of industrialization, and was often referred to as the modernization disease. The government expressed real concern about the effect that the increasing number of disabled people might be having on the economy and on society as a whole (Office of the Prime Minister, 1980, p. 1). In other words, the government sought to reduce its financial burden of caring for the disabled. Both medical and technological knowledge were employed in the 1970s in order to bring disabled people back into the workforce, as a valuable human resource for the industrialization and development era (1957–1987), and simultaneously to enhance both social and economic security.

This was a clear change in the Thai government's perception and treatment of disabled people. While they had been considered helpless or as disabled bodies during the nation-building era, in the new era of industrialization they were considered able-bodied and a potential resource that could be rehabilitated in order to join the manufacturing workforce. Through improvements in medical technology and rehabilitation techniques, people with disabilities were not only able to work and to look after themselves, but were also no longer seen as a burden on the state and their families (Office of the Prime Minister, 1980, p. 2).

During this period, the normalization medical model was applied to clarify the definition of disability, as well as to suggest approaches for prevention, treatment, and rehabilitation. For example, in 1976, a person with a disability was defined as 'a person with physical and/or mental impairment(s) who is unable to practice daily activities, study, and work as other people do' (Administrative and Legal Committee, 1976). The 1981 United Nations' declaration marking the International Year of Disabled Persons heralded a significant turning point in the Thai state's ideology and policies formulated with respect to people with disabilities. Following the UN declaration and influenced by the International Association of Persons with Disabilities as well as the World Health Organization, the Thai government produced a long-term plan for the rehabilitation of disabled people within four main areas: medicine, education, vocation, and society (Board of Event Organizers for International Year of Disabled Person, 1983, p. 113). Although each area was implemented differently, they shared the goal of ensuring that all disabled people became an active part of the industrialization process and could contribute to the development of the country, thus lowering the national economic and social burden. It is clear that while people with disabilities during the nation-building era had been regarded as obstacles to the formation of a civilized nation, during the industrialization era, people with disabilities were viewed as potential resources for economic growth.

Disability as a metaphor for moral disorder and urban problems

During the industrialization era, disability was divided into three categories: physical, mental, and social. No longer was disability the result of bad karma, but rather the result of various medical issues. Physical disability included visible physical disabilities and chronic illnesses resulting in some degree of body malfunction; mental disability included mental illness and intellectual retardation; and social disability included inappropriate and/ or abnormal behaviour, such as prostitution, begging, troublemaking, and crime. The government considered socially disabled people to be selfish, in that they created problems instead of being valuable members of the workforce and contributing to the economy (Social Welfare Division, 1983a, pp. 371-385).

As a result, social disability was seen as a symbol of social and moral disorder, particularly with regard to the social problems found in cities, and especially Bangkok. During this period, large numbers of people migrated from rural areas to Bangkok looking for work and a better life, and the government feared that these people, along with the disabled, would add to social problems in the city. Disabled people were often poor and uneducated, so the government assumed they would also be more likely to commit crimes and/or be more easily induced to commit violence (Theerabutrara, 1983, pp. 102–103). It might seem irrational to believe that disabled people would become big-city criminals, but this conclusion apparently reflected the inherited ideology of the time, that disabled people were vulnerable subjects.

During this period of rapid growth in Bangkok, people with disabilities were still placed in the same categories as the worst social and moral offenders: the homeless, beggars, and prostitutes. As a result, the Thai government established vocational training centres for people with disabilities in many provinces, in order to prevent rural disabled people from migrating to Bangkok and causing social problems and moral disorder (Social Welfare Division, 1983b, pp. 149–150).

At this time, disabilities were understood as medical conditions, and the government believed that advancements in medical technology and the effectiveness and efficiency of medical rehabilitation could restore disabled people to the ranks of the working and able-bodied. However, the Thai government encountered a significant obstacle when it tried to implement a long-term plan for people with disabilities: the lack of accurate data concerning the number of disabled people in Thailand. This lack of data was a product of the ideology inherited from the nation-building era, which viewed people with disabilities as ambiguous citizens—neither citizens nor non-citizens—and so not counted. In addition, there were no regulations in place for people with disabilities, making it difficult to direct the implementation of the plan (Board of Event Organizers for International Year of Disabled Persons, 1983, p. 120).

Thus, in the era of industrialization, while disabled people remained ambiguous, they were given the additional and contradictory baggage of being considered both human resources and citizens at risk of causing social problems, and, therefore, useless in terms of productivity. Their ambiguity was reinforced by the fact that they were still placed in the same category as the homeless, beggars, and prostitutes, meaning that they too should be confined to shelters, rehabilitation centres, and vocational training centres. What's more, the medical definition of disability as an individual tragedy continued to go hand-in-hand with the karma ideology of Theravada Buddhism. Disabled people living in this era embodied the contradiction between the karma doctrine's perception of the disabled body as an object waiting for assistance, and industrialization's demand for productive subjects. It is clear that the biopolitics practiced by the Thai state and contained within Theravada Buddhist beliefs were still intertwined and continued to reinforce one another, as would become manifest in 'the laws of compassion' introduced in the next decade.

Part II: The politics of compassion

In 1991, after almost two decades of preparation, the Thai state finally promulgated the Rehabilitation for Persons with Disabilities Act, the first law to define disabled people and their rights. The act was heavily influenced by the medical model of disability and a subsequent normalization of the medical rehabilitation approach. It defined a disabled person as 'a person with physical, intellectual, and mental impairment or abnormality' (Rehabilitation for Persons with Disabilities Act, 1991, pp. 18-28), thereby dropping the previous link between disability and social conditions.

Today, advocates for the disabled argue that the act and more recent legislation reflecting the humanitarian goals of Theravada Buddhism are equivalent to 'laws of compassion', which aim to provide charity rather than empower those with disabilities (Boontan, 2000, p. 65). Advocates for disabled people say that prejudice and discrimination towards people with disabilities must be combated through legislation that guarantees their civil rights (Institute of Health Promotion for People with Disability, 2008, pp. 34–37). After the military coup of 2006, the leaders of certain nongovernmental organizations (NGOs) working for disabled people— as members of policymaking committees during the drafting of a new constitution—proposed adding the word 'disability' to Section 30 of the new constitution to disallow social discrimination against people with disabilities (Institute of Health Promotion for People with Disability, 2007, p. 8). Watchara Riewpaiboon (1999, p. 27), a Thai scholar who has participated in the fight against discrimination towards disabled people, argues that advocates for disabled people realize, through experience, that only equitable laws will ensure equal rights for people with disabilities in Thai society. Their fight seemed to bear fruit—sixteen years later, the act was revised and presented as The Persons with Disabilities Empowerment Act, 2007.

This revised act, which was created through a social reform movement led by NGOs representing the rights of disabled people, is based on a politics of identity strategy and a human rights discourse, both of which were influenced by international organizations, especially the World Health Organization and the International Convention on the Rights of Persons with Disabilities. Activists emphasized that a social model of disability was important, not just because it highlighted what needed to be changed in terms of the barriers, prejudices, and discrimination faced by people with disabilities, but also because it provided the basis for a stronger sense of identity (Petkong, 2005). The 2007 act clearly reflects the international emphasis on the social model. For example, the new definition of persons with disabilities no longer implies physical abnormality, impairment, or disease as invoked by the medical model of disability, nor individual sin committed in a previous life as influenced by the karma ideology of Theravada Buddhism. Instead, the new definition relates to social dis-crimination and/or physical environmental barriers, those that impair or prevent disabled people from being able to live independently (Persons with Disabilities Empowerment Act, 2007, pp.8-24). However, based on the identity politics and human rights discourse, people with disabilities who look like beggars are ignored in the act of 2007 because they do not conform to the emancipatory agenda for disabled people in Thailand set by rights activists. For example, the Thai Association for the Blind has persuaded blind singers busking on street corners in Bangkok to sell lottery tickets, or to become traditional Thai massage therapists, with an aim of making them independent rather than begging and relying on philanthropy.

The ironies of the politics of identity

Although the politics of identity for disabled people in Thailand mainly aims to change the focus of the Thai government's ideology from the provision of charity to the protection of human rights, and from rehabilitation to empowerment, and although the movement seems to have had success driving forward new definitions under Thai law, I believe the political movement is ironic in and of itself. While trying to free disabled people of the state's limiting definitions, it has ended up reinforcing a categorization of disabled people that is based on a system of compulsory able-bodiedness, where being able-bodied means being capable of the normal physical exertions required in a particular system of labour (McRuer, 2006, p. 8). In addition, the movement reinforces the social model's dualism of impairment—which includes individual, physical and embodied experiences—and disability—which includes socially imposed disadvantages arising from cultural attitudes, the structural organization of institutions, and the design of public spaces (Corker, 1999).

I argue that the concept of impairment in Thailand is a construction of biopolitics, a historical legacy of Thai state ideology and biological discourse from each preceding era, reinforced by karmic doctrines and the rhetoric of compassion arising from Theravada Buddhism. Moreover, though the politics of identity strategy aims to create a collective identity for people with disabilities, it ends up conforming to the medical model, because what distinguishes the identity of such people from any other group is still their level of impairment. Inevitably, this aligns with the very medical model that the social model and human rights discourse attempt to counter (Bickenbach et al., 1999, p. 1182).

Conclusion

The social model for understanding disability is weak in that it regards an impaired body to be a neutral phenomenon, while disability is a social construction (see Abberley, 1987; Barnes, 1991; Oliver, 1990). There is no pure or natural body: the impaired body has no pre-social and historical existence free from biopolitics; it does not exist outside of discourses (Thomas,

1999; Tremain, 2002). On the contrary, impaired bodies are the product of both certain technologies of power and a biological discourse introduced by the modern Thai state, a product that conforms perfectly with institutional moralities drawn from Theravada Buddhism. Impairments are not only a biological fact, but also a discursive product, similar to the notion of sex. It is an effect rather than an origin, and a performance rather than an essence (see Haraway, 1991; Butler, 1993). For this reason, I also criticize the social model, which is strongly influenced by the historical-materialist philosophies of neo-Marxism, and which views power from the perspective of juridical conception—constructed as a fundamentally repressive force, and possessed by a centralized external authority such as a social group, a class, an institution, or a state, which reigns over others (Tremain, 2005, p. 9).

I argue instead for a post-structuralist approach, as influenced by the work of Foucault, who conceptualizes power not within individuals or social structures such as an institution, group, elite, or class in the historical-materialist sense of neo-Marxist philosophy, but instead operating in the everyday discourses of people (Foucault, 1978, 1982; Foucault and Gordon, 1980); it endeavours to control and monitor the social lives of people with impaired bodies, as has been the case on the modern Thai state era, in which contemporary biopower has left disabled people in the unenviable position of being considered 'ambiguous citizens'.

Acknowledgements

This article was enriched by the conversations and discussions I had with Professor Stuart Blume, and Professor Bernhard Hadolt also played a significant role revising and editing my text. I am also extremely grateful to the Ford Foundation in Thailand for granting me a doctoral fellowship for the research on which this article is based.

References

Abberley, P. (1987). The concept of oppression and the development of a social theory of disability. *Disability, Handicap & Society*, 2(1), 5–19.

Administrative and Legal Committee (1976). *Draft of Rehabilitation for Disabled People Act*. Mimeographed.

Agamben, G. (1998). *Homo sacer: Sovereign power and bare life*. D. Heller-Roazen, trans. Stanford: Stanford University Press.

Agamben, G. (2005). *State of Exception*. K. Attell, trans. Chicago: University of Chicago Press.

Barnes, C. (1991). *Disabled people in Britain and discrimination.* London: Hurst.

Bickenbach, J.E., Chatterji, S., Badley, E.M., and Üstün, T.B. (1999). Models of disablement, universalism and the ICIDH. *Social Science & Medicine, 48*(9), 1173–1187.

Board of Event Organizers for International Year of Disabled Persons (1983). National Plan of Social Work and Rehabilitation for Disabled People (1982–1991). In Department of Social Welfare, ed., *Document on International Year of Disabled Persons 1981* (pp. 110–121). Bangkok: Pimluk Press.

Boontan, M. (2000). Philosophy and Administrative Principle: In Association for the Blind People in Thailand. In M. Boontan, ed., *Three Decades of Association for the Blind People in Thailand.* Bangkok: Jirarat Print.

Butler, J. (1993). *Bodies that matter: On the discursive limits of sex.* London: Routledge.

Chotidilok, R. (1997). Madame La-iead Piboonsongkram and Her Establishment on Social Work in Thailand. In J. Panyarachun, ed., *Biography and Work of Madame La-iead Piboonsongkram.* Bangkok: Dansutha Print.

Corker, M. (1999). Differences, conflations and foundations: The limits to 'accurate', theoretical representation of disabled people's experience? *Disability and Society, 14*(5), 627–642.

Department of Social Welfare (1981). 41st anniversary of Department of Social Welfare [Special Issue]. *Social Welfare Magazine.* Nonthaburi: Pakgret Social Work Shelter for Women.

Department of Social Welfare (1990). *Fifty years of Department of Social Welfare* (pp. 102-103). Nonthaburi: Pakgret Social Work Shelter for Women Print.

Fassin, D. (2007). *When bodies remember: Experiences and politics of AIDS in South Africa.* A. Jacobs and G. Varro, trans. Berkeley: University of California Press.

Fassin, D. (2008). The embodied past: From paranoid style to politics of memory in South Africa. *Social Anthropology/Anthropologie Sociale, 16*(3), 312–328.

Foucault, M. (1978). *The history of sexuality. Vol. 1: An introduction.* R. Hurley, trans. New York: Vintage Books.

Foucault, M. (1982). The subject and power. In H.L. Dreyfus and P. Rabinow, eds., *Michel Foucault: Beyond structuralism and hermeneutics* (pp. 208–226). Chicago: University of Chicago Press.

Foucault, M., and Gordon, C., eds. (1980). *Power/knowledge: Selected interviews & other writings 1972–1977.* C. Gordon, L. Marshall, J. Mepham, and K. Soper, trans. New York: Pantheon Books.

Haraway, D. (1991). *Simians, cyborgs and women: The reinvention of nature.* London: Free Association Books.

Institute of Health Promotion for People with Disability (2007). *The Politics of Persons with Disabilities Newsletter, 4.*

Institute of Health Promotion for People with Disability (2008). *The Politics of Persons with Disabilities Newsletter, 13.*

Kasetsiri, C. (2008). *Thai Political History (1932-1957).* Bangkok: Social Science and Human Science Textbook Project Foundation.

Kawinraweekun, K. (2003). *Constructing the Body of Thai Citizens during the Phiboon Regime of 1938-1944.* Master Degree Thesis, Faculty of Sociology and Anthropology, Thammasat University.

McRuer, R. (2006). *Crip theory: Cultural signs of queerness and disability.* New York: New York University Press.

Office of the Prime Minister (1980). Announcement of International Year of Disabled Persons (1981) [Special issue]. *Royal Thai Government Gazette, 97*(162), 1–4.

Oliver, M. (1990). *The politics of disablement.* Basingstoke: Macmillan.

Persons with Disabilities Empowerment Act (2007). *Royal Thai Government Gazette, 124*(61A), 8–24.

Petkong, W. (2005). *The Civic Network of Disabled People: Identity Construction in Health System Reform Movement*. Nonthaburi: Society and Health Institute.

Poshakrishna, P. (1986). Madame La-iead Piboonsongkram: In the National Identity Office. In The National Identity Office, ed., *The Virtuous Women*. Bangkok: Secretary of the Prime Minister Office.

Prakitnonthakarn, C. (2009). *Arts and Architecture of the People's Party: Political Ideological Symbols*. Bangkok: Matichon Press.

Puaksom, D. (2007). *Germ, body and medicalised state: Modern medical history in Thailand.* Bangkok: Chulalongkorn University Press.

Rehabilitation for Persons with Disabilities Act [Special issue] (1991). *Royal Thai Government Gazette,108*(205), 18–28.

Riewpaiboon, W. (1999). *The literature review for service system development and rehabilitation in order to improve the quality of life of disabled people*. Bangkok: Health System Research Institute.

Riewpaiboon, W., and Blume, S. (2009). Disability and rehabilitation in Europe and North America: Disability and rehabilitation in Asia. In R. Addlakha, S. Blume, P. Devlieger, O. Nagase, and M. Winance, eds., *Disability and society: A reader* (p. xvii-xxv). New Delhi: Orient Black Swan.

Rose, N., and Novas, C. (2005). Biological citizenship. In A. Ong and S. Collier, eds.,*Global assemblages: Technology, politics and ethics as anthropological problems* (pp. 439–463). Malden: Blackwell Publishing.

Social Welfare Division (1983a). Disabled people and rehabilitation. In Department of Social Welfare, ed., *Document on International Year of Disabled Persons 1981* (pp. 371–385). Bangkok: Pimluk Press.

Social Welfare Division (1983b). Administration on Social Work and Rehabilitation for Disabled People. In Department of Social Welfare, ed., *Document on International Year of Disabled Persons 1981* (pp. 141–155). Bangkok: Pimluk Press.

Suwannathat–Pian, K. (1995). *Thailand's Durable Premier: Phibun through Three Decades 1932–1957*. New York: Oxford University Press.

Theerabutrara, S. (1983). Problem of disabled people in City and Social Welfare Council. In Department of Social Welfare, ed., *Document on International Year of Disabled Persons 1981* (pp. 98–115). Bangkok: Pimluk Press.

Thomas, C. (1999). *Female forms: Experiencing and understanding disability*. Buckingham: Open University Press.

Tremain, S. (2002). On the subject of impairment. In M. Corker and T. Shakespeare, eds., *Disability/postmodernity: Embodying political theory* (pp. 32–47). London: Continuum Press.

Tremain, S. (2005). Foucault, governmentality, and critical disability theory: An introduction. In S. Tremain, ed., *Foucault and the government of disability* (pp. 1–24). Ann Arbor: University of Michigan Press.

Vajanasara, K. (2005). *Social representation of disabled people in Thailand: A case study of Thai literatures*. Nonthaburi: The Health Promotion for People with Disability in Thailand Program, Health System Research Institute, Thai Health Promotion Foundation, and Sirindhorn National Medical Rehabilitation Centre.

5 Market thinking and home nursing

Perspectives on new socialities in healthcare in Denmark

Bodil Ludvigsen

Some months after the launch of a new management system to manage and plan the workload of a group of Danish home nurses, a home nurse was talking about the impact of changes on her work processes:

> Work continuity is not the same anymore and it's a shame. Actually it takes the pleasure out of one's job. The problem is that one day I will be visiting some patients and the next day I don't really know what is happening, because others are visiting them instead. It's a real shame.

She went on to talk about her lack of personal knowledge about the patients and the fact that she was no longer able to follow up on their care:

> Today, say—I had perhaps four new patients. It's simply not very good, because you can't really follow up on much, although we have to write everything down for the nurses who come the next few days. I don't initiate many things either, because I don't know anything about the patient. For example, I can't see if her legs have been swollen for some time, or if her legs are less swollen because of the medicine. So, I'm just a tool, who comes and administers the pills.

Introduction

During my fieldwork among elderly people receiving home nursing,[1] a new informational technology (IT) system was introduced in the planning of

---

1   Home nursing in Denmark is a legal right for all citizens and free of charge according to the Danish Health Care Act, on the condition that general practitioners, hospitals, specialists, or others request home nursing for the specific citizen. Local municipalities are financially responsible for the home nurse organizations as to level of service, for example, when the home nurses' visits are to take place—day, evening, and/or night; how many visits and for how long; and what kind of home nursing the recipient needs. Home nursing is supposed to treat and nurse citizens in their own homes, prevent hospital admittance, facilitate daily living, and postpone elderly people's need of nursing homes. It also is supposed to provide support

home nursing. This new system pooled the names of all nurses and patients who were due to receive a visit each day, and distributed the patients among the nurses, mainly depending on the daily workload of each nurse. This was a more random way of distributing patients and tasks, as the personal knowledge of patients and nurses counted less. Previously, small groups of nurses worked together in districts where they jointly planned and implemented home nursing for citizens living in the district who needed nursing care and treatment. Organized this way, patients and nurses came to know each other relatively well. The introduction of the new system, however, meant that nurses visited more patients they did not know, and this influenced the manners through which patients and nurses created social relations with each other, as well as the opportunities nurses had to follow up on patients' progress. The new IT system drew my attention to how system change affected elderly people and their nurses. It seemed that organizational changes influenced the opportunities elderly people and nurses had to create and maintain social relationships with each other in multiple ways. In addition, the elderly people often talked about the worrisome constant replacement of staff, and how they preferred dealing with people they already knew.

Changes to the ways home nursing was organized had its origin in a marketization process that started back in the 1990s when management methods and market principles and thinking were first introduced into the Danish National Health Service (Sehested, 2002; Knudsen, 2007), and which since has gradually developed. Within home nursing, competition and free choice is now a reality: 6% of Danish citizens who receive personal care and 48% of those who receive practical help in managing their homes receive this service through private companies (Ministry of Social Affairs and Integration, 2012), although it is paid for by local councils. Danish councils can legally outsource home nursing, but so far only one council has outsourced this service.

Prior to the introduction of the new IT system, home nurses, as health professionals, largely managed their workload independently. However, central and local politicians had for some years requested greater transparency regarding, insight into, and control of home nurses' work and effectiveness,

---

in administering medication and dressing wounds, palliative care, care of the chronically ill, and illness prevention. Finally, home nursing is charged with the guidance, supervision, and planning of nursing care around the clock after discharge from hospital, and educating patients, relatives, and staff members. Home nurses collaborate with home helpers, general practitioners, hospitals, hospices, pharmacies, and relatives, among others.

as well as the performance of other public employees. The IT system allowed this to take place within home nursing and the localized group and nurse-managed organizational system were transformed into a centralized system. It facilitated the central distribution of home nursing visits, and increased the likelihood of daily replacement of nurses. Consequently, continuity diminished and longer intervals between visits by the same nurse became more common.

In this contribution I examine the impact on relationships and interactions between elderly people and their home nurses when management and market thinking dominate and organizational systems change. I ask: Do changes to the guiding principle have implications for home nursing and for the elderly, and if so, what are the consequences for social relations? I want to shed light on how changes to the daily management of nurses' workload affect social relations between elderly people and their nurses.

Methods and informants

This study is part of the Centre for Healthy Aging, Programme 4, which focuses on society, culture, and preventive medicine.[2] The findings discussed here are based on anthropological fieldwork in a local council near Copenhagen, where I followed, interviewed, and carried out participant observation with fifteen elderly people. I met my informants, aged 58–95 years (average 86), on between two and eight occasions (on average five times) over a period of six to eighteen months. I also interviewed another nine elderly patients one time each. The fieldwork ended in July 2011. The study focused on elderly people's medication, health activities, everyday life, social relations, who influenced their health concerns, and their adaptation to changing life circumstances.

All the participating elderly people received home nursing for their medication, and their home nurses enabled me to contact them in their homes. Establishing contact with this 'hard to reach' group of elderly people would

---

2   The Centre for Healthy Aging focuses on research into aging for better health and reduced frailty throughout life. The five multidisciplinary programmes investigate biomedical, social, and psychological causes of healthy aging. Programme 4, 'Society and Culture: Health Care Policy and Preventive Medicine', focuses on the analysis of health policies, organization of the healthcare system, and medical technologies available for use in preventive medication. The centre started its activities in January 2009; it is administratively placed under the Faculty of Health Sciences, University of Copenhagen, and was established through a donation from Nordea-fonden to the University of Copenhagen. See: http://healthyaging.ku.dk/.

have been difficult without assistance, as many spent most of their time at home, and when going out they generally visited family or neighbours, or went shopping. Few visited day-care centres or other organizations. Therefore, an introduction by a trusted person (as home nurses explicitly were) was needed to facilitate appointments; furthermore, quite a few were unable to leave their home without assistance. None of the informants were memory impaired, but many were frail and facing several diagnoses, some quite serious. The fieldwork also included interviews with home nurses, participant observation of their home visits to other citizens, and interviews with relatives of elderly informants.

Theoretical background

The English linguist Norman Fairclough (1992) has developed a method of critical discourse analysis based on analyses of language in social practices, and he finds that discourses help constitute social identities, social relations, and knowledge—and meaning systems.

> Discourses do not just reflect or represent social entities and relations, they construct or 'constitute' them; different discourses constitute key entities (be they 'mental illness', 'citizenship' or 'literacy') in different ways, and position people in different ways as social subjects (e.g. as doctors or patients), and it is these social effects of discourse that are focused upon in discourse analysis. (Fairclough, 1992, p. 3ff.)

In many countries in recent years there has been an upsurge in the extension of the market to new areas of social life. According to Fairclough (1992, p. 207), a commodification process can emerge in institutions and social domains—even those who do not produce commodities in the narrow economic sense of goods for sale—in which they become organized and understood as producing goods and products to be delivered. Sectors with a focus on education, healthcare, and the arts have, for example, restructured and reconceptualized their activities as the production of goods for customers, and people working in these sectors have reconstructed and re-established perceptions of their activities, social relations, and social and professional identities due to changes in discourse practices, such as the use of language (Fairclough, 1992, p. 6). Fairclough points to the 'rewording' of activities and communities, such as students being referred to as 'consumers' or 'clients', and educational courses as 'packages' or 'products'.

These areas are 'colonized' by types of discourses derived from advertising, management, and counselling (Fairclough, 1992, p. 7).

This process has increasingly resulted in the extension of the market in the Danish healthcare sector, where health and care activities have been re-structured and reconceptualized. As in the education sector, the healthcare sector produces 'packages', another word for professional performances, which are rendered to 'customers', as patients may be called. What remains to be established is whether patients' and healthcare workers' socialities change due to such discursive and organizational changes.

The American sociologist Viviana Zelizer asks in her book *The Purchase of Intimacy* (2005, p. 3): 'Does the penetration of an ever-expanding market threaten intimate social life?' She rejects the argument made by critics, philosophers, and politicians, who all insist, as she puts it: 'that public policy must insulate household relations, personal care, and love itself, from an invading, predatory, economic world', arguing that everyone uses 'economic activity to create, maintain, and renegotiate important ties' (Zelizer, 2005, p. 3). The balance between the household and other areas is, according to Zelizer, not easy to uphold, but if disputes arise, it is certain that new definitions of behaviour in different social relations come into play. In 1994, Zelizer published the book *The Social Meaning of Money*, which illustrated how money affects people's social relationships, showing that social practices between people did change with the expansion of monetary transactions in American society, and that people not only incorporated money into the construction of new social ties, but also transformed its meaning when doing so (Zelizer, 2005, p. 2).

Zelizer's (2005, p. 15) use of 'intimate relations' covers a range of relation-ships between children and parents, spouses, siblings, and friends, but also between patients and their therapists, traders and their customers, as well as lawyers, coaches, vicars, or others in different relationships. Zelizer points to nurses' work, which seen from their employers' point of view, is successful if they carry out their nursing tasks well, get patients to follow treatments, respond to patients' symptoms or life-threatening situations, and prevent complaints (Zelizer, 2005, p. 187). Achieving this, she argues, requires that 'nurses establish close relations with their charges. Not only do they provide intimate bodily and emotional attention, but they also deploy the skilled practices of personal intimacy—joking, cajoling, consoling, and sympathetic listening' (Zelizer, 2005, p. 187).

My fieldwork showed that elderly people and their nurses did negotiate as Zelizer documents—not over monetary issues but tasks and time, an equivalent to money. During the process of exchanging viewpoints and ideas, negotiations and renegotiations, and not least by being together when doing so, the elderly people and the nurses often created social relations. Locating Fairclough and Zelizer side by side brings two different perspectives into play as both researchers, among other things, are looking at the process of marketization, outcomes, and socialities.

Market thinking in the public sector

Changes in legislation and management methods have altered the Danish healthcare system from a relatively independently and professionally based system, to a system where competition, market thinking, and management approaches play a growing role. Patients in need of hospital treatment and home help can now choose between service providers, but people over 80 years of age seldom chose these opportunities,[3] and the elderly people in my fieldwork certainly preferred the public service. As a result of the rise of market thinking within the public sector, even though outsourcing was rarely used, employees faced issues regarding efficiency, standardization, and evaluation (Sehested, 2002, p. 1519), and had to document the number of daily visits and time spent on each task. On the other hand, the Danish healthcare legislation[4] is built on easy and equal access, quality, and professionalism, and home nursing is a citizen's right—a right that in its essence is ethical, following anthropologists Sharon Kaufman and Lakshmi Fjord (2010, p. 412), who argue that Medicare is an ethical programme for elderly Americans.

To some extent, the basic concept of healthcare as ethical, with equal access for all, stands in contrast to market principles and economic requirements, and this has gradually produced conflicting agendas for healthcare professionals. As discussed in the introduction, the home nurse met several new patients every day, and experienced difficulties in following up on their

3   Please see: 'Frit valg i ældreplejen' (2011), pp. 14–15, http://www.kora.dk/media/277495/ RAPPORT_Frit_valg_i_aeldreplejen.pdf (last accessed: 22 February 2014).

4   The first two paragraphs in the Danish Health Care Act read: '§ 1 Healthcare aims to promote public health and to prevent and treat disease, suffering and disability for the individual. § 2 The Act lays down requirements for health care in order to ensure respect for the individual, its integrity and self-determination and to meet the need for (1) easy and equal access to health care, (2) high-quality treatment, (3) correspondence between benefits, (4) freedom of choice, (5) easy access to information, (6) a transparent healthcare system, and 7) short waiting time'. See: https://www.retsinformation.dk/forms/r0710.aspx?id=130455#K1 (last accessed: 18 March 2013).

cases and hence being as professional as she expected herself to be. For the home nurse the conflicting agendas were (1) the professional and ethical obligations to take the health needs, social conditions, and individual understandings of the elderly into consideration, and (2) management responsibilities, including conforming to and following standard procedures and documenting time spent.

Economic demands, efficiency, and market thinking has left its mark on the Danish public sector (Knudsen, 2007), and the introduction of the concept of free choice has changed the rhetoric. The rewording process, as Fairclough claims (1992, p. 207), was to some extent observed within the home-nursing sector, where in recent years key professional tasks in home nursing were referred to as 'services'. Also the rhetorical use of the term 'patient' has been subject to change. At present, he or she is referred to as a 'citizen', 'client', or 'user' (the words are directly translated from Danish). In common terminology most Danish councils and home nurses referred to inhabitants and patients as 'citizens'. Nevertheless, on occasion nurses would, with some sarcasm, refer to citizens as 'our customers'. This indicated a change of rhetoric and perhaps a shift in thinking, as Fairclough suggests. In relation to the interplay between economics, social relations, and emotions, Zelizer highlights the negotiations that take place between the different parties. My argument is that negotiations continue to take place between elderly and professional staff, on the condition that the elderly have the strength and the opportunity to do so, but also that social relations change if managing and organizing principles do not maintain the opportunity for the elderly and the professionals to meet on a regular basis.

How does it work? Creating social relations between elderly people and home nurses

Home nurses drew attention to the fact that good social relations facilitated the nursing process and consequently that nursing tasks could be performed more smoothly for the elderly and the nurse. The elderly people and home nurses created social relations or 'relatedness' when nurses visited the elderly people in their homes, over a shorter or longer period of time, while they talked, listened, shared experiences, gave advice, touched, and performed individual nursing care for the elderly (Ludvigsen, 2006). Relatedness is a concept developed by anthropologist Janet Carsten during her fieldwork with a Malaysian family in the 1980s (1995). In her later work Carsten (2000, 2004) describes how relatedness develops in chosen families, among friends, in neighbourhoods, and other places. It is established and developed when people are together in the same place, sharing and perform-ing activities, tasks, or processes together over a period of time. In a previous study (Ludvigsen, 2006) I suggested that the concept of relatedness is also useful in a professional setting, such as home nursing. This is the case even though family activities tend to be of a more intimate nature, such as eating together; living in the same place; sharing resources, possessions, and effects; and sharing experiences, good or bad, and events with each other. While home nurses never ate with the elderly and rarely drank a cup of coffee, they might still share good as well as bad health and life experiences with the elderly people, and they provided useful nursing equipment for the elderly, such as medicine boxes, dressing materials, and assistive devices.

Social relations between the elderly and the nurses were essentially professional and personal, but not private. A professional and personal relationship, as I saw it performed, is characterized by professionals showing an interest, respect, and kindness, for example, asking how a celebration went or referencing other points of conversation from a previous visit. This took place at the same time as dialogues, consultations, and negotiations, as Zelizer points out, of what was necessary for the patient. The nurse shared who she/he was as a person, mostly that he/she was trustworthy, but generally the nurses' own problems, private matters, economics, politics, and religion were not discussed. The elderly on the other hand, revealed private information simply by being in a position of needing assistance, as home nurses' access to the homes of the elderly transfers information about homes and residents, through their appearance (e.g. tidiness, messiness, dirt, odours) and the presence of photos and other objects, in addition to health matters. But how can nurses utilize this information and make use of established relationships if they, due to the new organizational system, do not see the elderly for a period of time? How does this change influence their socialities? Would nurses and patients become accustomed to a more superficial kind of relationship in the home-nursing process if nurses were unable to utilize knowledge about a patient and establish social relations and relatedness?

Barriers might hinder some relationships, while social relations may be established immediately for others. This applied to the elderly and home nurses as well, though none were able to identify the specific reason. How-ever, both indicated that the first nurse who visited the elderly often was the person the elderly person related to best, and vice versa. Nurses stated that they generally prepared themselves for the first meeting with a new patient by being neutral and receptive in order to facilitate the process. It was not a given that the same nurse returned in the following days. Nurses did, however, adapt to the new system, which not only directed their activities in new ways and but also imposed a new hegemonic discourse based on the extension of the market process.

The elderly people who received visits from the home nurse for the first time were often just discharged from hospital and knew neither the person who came to nurse them, nor the purpose or what to expect. Hence, the first meeting was important and home nurses allowed extra time in order to become acquainted with the patient and to enable a dialogue that balanced what the patient wanted and what could be rendered. Most elderly people said that they deliberately met professionals in a friendly way. According to both, prolonged and repeated contact generally led to closer and more trustful relationships, as they got to know each other's positions from previous negotiations and dialogues, and could proceed from there. Through dialogue, small talk, physical proximity, and touch, for example, when nurses carried out treatments, injections, and changed dressings, the elderly and the nurses developed a kind of intimacy, learning from each other's reactions what could be spoken about and what could not. The home nurses and the patients were both aware that nursing needs decided the length of their relationship, and both stated that continuity in the social relations was preferential, that is, if they were on good terms. However, the duration of different nursing activities, such as the administration of medicine, was often a subject of negotiations between the elderly and their home nurses.

Essentially, home nurses' overall objective was to strengthen the elderly and enable them to manage by themselves. This underlying aim highlights the fragility of the relationship, however much valued, as some elderly expressed. Several of the elderly feared they might be required to manage their medicine on their own. Others valued being independent and free from visits, while still appreciating having the option for home nursing if their health grew weaker again. Sometimes home nurses were confronted with their loyalty to professional standards, which could not be followed meticulously in all homes. My research into home nursing and other researchers' reproduction of historical narratives about home nursing show that out of necessity home nurses are used to adapting professional standards to the reality in people's homes (Ludvigsen, 2006; Uhrenfeldt, 2001, p. 118).

Nurses were accustomed to negotiating with the elderly with regard to elderly people's self-determination, and nurses attempted to promote health by informing and giving advice with a readiness to compromise. One patient, for example, had been living with diabetes for many years and was fully aware that his food consumption did not match the recommended diabetic diet. In this case the nurse postponed talking about diet and focused on the patient's total well-being instead. If, however, the patient had a new diagnosis of diabetes, the nurse would advise and follow up on diet. Changing people's habits and living conditions was difficult to deal with and sometimes the nurse's intentions were not achievable in the short term, thus requiring negotiations and renegotiations over a longer period.

New management principles resulted in longer intervals between visits by the same nurse, a fact that did not contribute to creating and maintaining social relations and relatedness, as relationships were built by being together in the same place over a period of time while performing mutual activities (Carsten, 1995). These adjustments made the professional task more difficult for the nurses, in terms of providing individual advice, information, and treatment, and in providing nursing care. Nurses could not monitor the elderly, their illnesses, treatment, and general health as closely as previously. The question is whether the introduction of new management principles and market thinking into an organization leads to unforeseen consequences in the short or long run, as Fairclough suggests, or whether, as Zelizer argues, people always negotiate such relationships.

An organizational study of sales work under a marketization and competition process showed that it had implications for social relations exposed to marketization. The study examined key social relations of sales workers on two sites and the relationships constituted by monetary transactions. The authors summarize their findings: 'one group of workers is enmeshed in a dehumanised, instrumental and antagonistic set of relations, while another, smaller, group of workers is insulated against such relations by the functioning of tight trust based referral networks' (Korczynski and Ott, 2005, p. 707). The authors concluded that social relations in this kind of market situation were influenced by the social composition and constitution of the specific product market in which workers acted (Korczynski and Ott, 2005, p. 726). The marketization process seemed to erode the factors that supported the relations of trust-based networks, pointing to the importance of understanding the social nature of the workplace. In the home nurse organization these matters were not at play to the same degree. Nevertheless, the social nature of the workplace was undergoing a transformation, as the implementation of new ways of managing workload did not sustain either the continuity or the creation of social relations, which were central and valuable for both nurses and the elderly.

Elderly people in the light of social relations, socialities, and prevailing market thinking

Historically and culturally, the elderly people in this study lived their child-hood in the early stages of the Danish welfare state and their adult life during the unfolding phase of the welfare system in the 1960s and 1970s. Generally they expressed their loyalty to the system and many were grateful for the assistance. The common attitude to material goods was characterized by modesty: 'I've got what I need.' Many of the elderly were reluctant to use private hospitals, for example, for surgery, or private companies for cleaning, even though these were paid for by the welfare system. The elderly people in this study explicitly preferred help provided by the local council and not private companies: 'I've thought about it, but they are certainly not better, and I prefer the council, which I know', was a common statement. This finding was consistent with the analysis by the Dutch philosophers Andries Baart et al. (2008) of care of very old people in Western societies. The authors drew attention to a difference between people between 65 and 80 and the very old (more than 80 years old). According to Baart et al., the older group needed more help as they were less likely to be in a good shape, energetic, self-confident, and independent, with a purposeful understanding of their life project: 'The very old do not fit into the scheme of autonomous and self-conscious clients, who buy the care and cure they wish to be given. The very old do not fit into the autonomous model of human existence, with its concurrent claims about freedom of choice and the unencumbered self' (Baart et al., 2008, p. 22). The socialities of the elderly in my study did not change, as they remained loyal to the professional assistance they received from the council.

Several elderly people in my study also revealed that around the age of 80, they experienced a change in their health, becoming more fragile and dependent on treatment, care, and other public services; this change in their health limited their independence. According to Baart et al. (2008, p. 24) this fragility is in general kept out of everybody's sight as long as possible. A number of studies show how old people value their independence (see, for example, Leeson, 2001), and how a wish for independence is expressed at both individual and societal level: 'The ideal citizen is one who acts responsibly, is strong-willed, and acknowledges that he or she plays the essential role in solving his or her own problems' (Mik-Meyer and Villadsen, 2013, p. 4). In this respect the elderly people were ideal citizens. They tried to solve their problems and expressed a hope of managing on their own with the help of the council, and hence staying as autonomous as possible for as long as possible, by learning to adapt to physical impairment. However, they did not seem to adapt to discourses about the prevailing marketization and free choice in the manner Fairclough suggests. Nevertheless, the elderly people did to some extent negotiate conditions, as Zelizer claims, by asking for assistance from the council.

Despite the negative effects of aging, by ill health or disabilities, or in the aftermath of such, which restricted their mobility or caused pain and discomfort, the elderly considered themselves full members of society. By voting in elections or commenting on political debates at the local and national level elderly people enacted their role as members of society. They spoke of themselves as senior citizens who led a relatively independent life. Receiving assistance from home helpers,[5] assistive devices, and care from home nurses made it easier to live independently without having to rely on family. Not wanting to be a nuisance or inconvenience to their family was an all-encompassing wish (see, for example, Rostgaard, 2009). While the elderly were well aware of their age, they still felt they were the same person they were in their youth, albeit now with life experience. On the other hand, several of the elderly people noted that they were often looked upon as being elderly. In meetings with professionals, the elderly talked about being overlooked if other people were involved in the medical visit. Such experiences made them feel offended and worthless. They usually did not experience this attitude with people face-to-face, or with those they had social relations, such as their home nurses.

If the elderly criticized the help they received it was usually targeted at distant leaders, hospitals, and politicians. Typically, the elderly disapproved of the continuous replacement of staff, especially their favourite ones, and criticism regarding the lack of continuity gradually increased following the management change from local nursing districts to a centralized system. From this perspective the elderly people were attached to their established social relations and socialities, and did not want to change.

---

5   'Home help' is the common phrase describing that the municipal council is obliged to offer, and includes (i) personal care and assistance; (ii) assistance or support for necessary practical activities in the home; and (iii) meals services. Such assistance shall be offered to persons who are unable to carry out these activities due to temporary or permanent impairment of physical or mental function or special social problems. See: http://sm.dk/en/files/consolidation-act-on-social-services-1.pdf, part 16.

Closing remarks

In this article I have shown that the relationship between elderly people and home nurses did not change initially, as both the elderly and the nurses were anchored in a specific way of thinking and in their socialities—the elderly as citizens and nurses as professionals. However, both felt a change in the daily work. While the many different nurses visiting the elderly and the frequent change of personnel were a continuous concern for the elderly, they nevertheless expressed loyalty and trust in the public system and staff. However, frustrated and displeased comments became more frequent during my fieldwork, but remained within an understanding of the public system as public; they did not view the help they received as a commodity or the managing system as a commercial way of providing help. Free choice was not a preferred alternative for elderly people over 80 years old. They preferred receiving help from the council, despite the fact that the elderly did not know who was arriving at what time or how the tasks would be performed. In the light of everybody's outspoken wish for continuity and for visits by the same person, the increasing number of visits by different nurses and home helpers were noticeable.

The nurses, from their perspective, were not able to follow up on elderly people's health, progress, or decline in the same way as prior to the managerial changes. They voiced disapproval about changes to the managing system, as their influence over whom they would visit was reduced. The majority of nurses acknowledged the lack of continuity and hence the weaknesses of the system, however, they still accepted the system.

I have also shown that negotiations took place (Zelizer, 2005) between elderly people and professional staff. The elderly and home nurses regularly discussed upcoming tasks and times of future visits, as they had always done, but the system change implied that these negotiations now took place between different nurses, rather than between the elderly and a regular nurse. Such changes are likely to reduce the ability of the elderly to have their voice heard, as nurses and other professionals are less familiar with the elderly and their needs.

A preliminary conclusion suggests that market thinking, introduced by organizational changes in the form of a new IT system, conveys changes similar to those Fairclough pointed out. Nursing may in this case be understood as a kind of product to be delivered. Furthermore, the possibility of developing and maintaining social relations and relatedness between elderly people and nurses altered due to the features of the IT system. Consequently, changes in social relations are a likely outcome when managing and organizing principles do not support regular interactions between elderly people and professionals. Instead of maintaining continuity, the purpose of the system was to make the workload visible. Socialities were not necessarily changed by the introduction of management and market thinking per se, but were highly influenced by the social constructs of the workplace, as the work of Korczynski and Ott (2005) also showed.

An 80-year-old man described the rapid change of professionals following the introduction of the new organizational system: 'For a long time there were no problems, but now they change staff all the time. Initially there were four home nurses, who came here, and they were all very nice—at the moment a lot more nurses come. They have changed it [the system], and they have done it for their own sake, not for the sake of patients. That's for certain.'

References

Baart, A., Vosman, J., and Frans, J.H. (2008). Being witness to the lives of the very old. *Sociale Inventie*, *17*(3), 21–32.

Carsten, J. (1995). The substance of kinship and the heat of the hearth, feeding, personhood, and relatedness among Malays in Palau Langkawi. *American Ethnologist*, *22*(2), 223–239.

Carsten, J. (2000). *Cultures of relatedness.* Cambridge: Cambridge University Press.

Carsten, J. (2004). *After kinship.* Cambridge: Cambridge University Press.

Fairclough, N. (1992). *Discourse and social change.* Cambridge: Cambridge University Press.

Kaufman, S.R., and Fjord, L. (2011). Medicare, ethics, and reflexive longevity: Governing time and treatment in an aging society. *Medical Anthropology Quarterly*, *25*(2), 209–231.

Knudsen, T. (2007). *Fra folkestyre til markedsdemokrati: Dansk demokratihistorie efter 1973.* Copenhagen: Akademisk Forlag.

Korczynski, M., and Ott, U. (2005). Sales work under marketization: The social relations of the cash nexus? *Organization Studies*, *26*(5), 707–728.

Leeson, G.W. (2001). *New horizons—new elderly: The Danish longitudinal future study.* Copenhagen: Dane Age.

Ludvigsen, B. (2006). *Hvad er det med de sociale relationer I hjemmesygeplejen?* Unpublished master's thesis. University of Copenhagen, Copenhagen, Denmark.

Mik-Meyer, N., and Villadsen, K. (2013). *Power and welfare: Understanding citizens' encounters with state welfare.* London: Routledge.

Rostgaard, T. (2009). Dansk ældrepleje I et nordisk og europæisk perspektiv. In S. Glasdam and B.A. Esbensen, eds., *I Gerontologi–Livet som ældre i et moderne samfund* (pp. 61–75). Copenhagen: Nyt Nordisk Forlag, Arnold Busck.

Sehested, K. (2002). How new public management reforms challenge the roles of professionals. *International Journal of Public Administration*, *25*(12), 1513–1537.

Uhrenfeldt, L. (2001). Fra barmhjertighed til sundhedsfremme—træk af hjemmesygeplejens historiske udvikling i Danmark. In E.S. Nielsen and K. Lomborg, eds., *På arbejde i hjemmet: En bog om hjemmepleje* (pp. 113–133). Copenhagen: Gyldendal.

Zelizer, V.A. (2005). *The purchase of intimacy.* Princeton: Princeton University Press.

6 The production and transformation of subjectivity

Healthcare and migration in the province of Bologna (Italy)

Ivo Quaranta

Subjectivity: On power and agency

The concept of subjectivity has re-emerged in anthropology as a way to come back to the relationship of the mutual construction of personal and collective processes, with specific attention to the issue of power. On the one hand, the concept is engaged to 'consider how far subjectivities are determined by discourses, political economy, state structures, and personal dispositions [...] beyond the analytic limits of individualism and the lone heroic actor' (Werbner, 2002, p. 3). On the other hand, the concept is invoked to raise questions about agency and the possibility of social actors to negotiate the terms of their existence (Moore, 2007; Ortner, 2006). As Judith Butler (1997, p. 2) puts it: '[I]f, following Foucault, we understand power as *forming* the subject as well, as providing the very condition of its existence and the trajectory of its desire, then power is not simply what we oppose but also, in a strong sense, what we depend on for our existence and what we harbor and preserve in the beings that we are.'

The renewed anthropological focus on subjectivity has been framed as an attempt to ethnographically ground biopolitical processes, avoiding the theoretical consideration of power as a meta-empirical domain rooted in discourses rather than in practices and experience. Within such a framework, many authors have looked to the work of Giorgio Agamben (1998, 2005) and the concept of bare life in order to problematize the institutional dynamics related to policies aimed at safeguarding, promoting, and caring for human life (in both health and illness).[1]

The global and local dynamics linked to the contemporary economic and financial crisis, coupled with an increasingly market-based approach to health and social care merely concerned with cost reduction, have contributed to

---

[1] Giorgio Agamben, by retrieving Walter Benjamin's expression, has claimed that today all politics is biopolitics in so far as the definition of life in terms of biological existence (devoid of personal and social qualification) has become the mark of ordinary forms of sovereignty.

limit health systems in their capacity to respond to the right to health, thus reducing its attainability. It is against this background that the concept of biological citizenship (as theorized by Adriana Petryna (2002) and Nikolas Rose and Carlos Novas (2005), among many others) can help us to focus on the very processes that construct subjects as bearers of rights and responsibilities around specific biopolitical predicaments. This line of reasoning has been widely adopted in the context of humanitarian intervention (Fassin, 2010; Fassin and Pandolfi, 2010; Nguyen, 2005); however, it can also be applied to the case of economic and political migrants, whose possibility of claiming fundamental rights is often tied to specific biological conditions (Ticktin, 2011).

Asylum seekers, people living in extreme marginality, economic migrants, and others who are not granted citizenship often end up trapped in the institutional construction of the suffering body as the residual ground on which to claim access to state services (Fassin, 2001a, p. 5). As Vinh-Kim Nguyen (2006, p. 71) states: 'as ever steeper gradients of social inequality register in the bodies of the poor, their fates are increasingly tied to their biology and the politics of intervening on it'. The complicated system of assistance to migrants appears to be centred on the production of specific kinds of subjectivity. In the Italian context, 'autonomy', 'responsibility', and 'emancipation' are the keywords around which assistance programmes organize their support services, through teaching and training workshops, in the attempt to forge proper subjects: in other words, good workers, responsible carers and parents, fluent Italian speakers, and diligent citizens (Ong, 2003).

The contemporary focus on subjectivity aims, however, not only at investigating the social construction of inner personal processes, but also at analysing the ways through which such processes give birth to specific forms of agency. On the one hand, it is within such biopolitical dynamics that marginalized immigrant people in Italy become subjects and can access resources they are otherwise denied; on the other hand, within the same processes unexpected forms of action can emerge, imposing the need to problematize the very concept of agency (Comaroff, 2006). Didier Fassin (2000) suggests theorizing the relationship between *bare life* and *forms of life*, in order to go beyond the opposition between subject and power. In this sense, the identity politics approach and the biopolitical one are not mutually exclusive (Whyte, 2009). They can—and should—be carried out together, exploring the relationship and the transformative tension existing between bare life and forms of life; agency, in fact, can take place from within biopower. In the following pages I argue that agency can be understood in terms of actors' capability to critically engage the processes of their own construction/constriction.

The experience of the Socio-Cultural Consultation Centre in the province of Bologna: Theoretical orientation and methodological choices

The reflections presented in this paper arise from work done at the Socio-Cultural Consultation Centre for Migrants' Health (CCC) since 2009, in the province of Bologna. The CCC was established as part of the provincial socio-sanitary plan, with the aim of providing consultation to professionals in the health and social services experiencing (relational) problems while attending to foreign patients. The CCC works through a multidisciplinary and multimethod approach, thanks to the involvement of anthropologists (like myself), public health professionals, social workers, ethnopsychiatrists, and psychologists, all with previous work or research experience with migrants. Established at the end of 2009, the first twelve months of activity were dedicated to meetings with professionals of the local health and social services in order to illustrate the CCC's features and functioning. In the following years, over 40 cases were referred for consultation (nine of them required an in-depth involvement with patients, whereas the other ones required only a consultation with the professionals in charge of the cases).

The first step of the consultation process investigates the needs of the unit(s) that activated the CCC, and documents how the professionals involved have framed the problem, what has already been done, and what they consider to be problematic in dealing with the patient. Depending on the key elements that emerge at this preliminary stage, a team is formed among the CCC's staff. The team is then in charge of the entire consultation process, reporting to the broader group during weekly meetings for general discussion and evaluation.

The second step is centred on consultation with the patient. This phase usually involves several encounters, including (when needed and agreed upon) the patient's significant others (family members, friends, others who may be relevant for dealing with the case). Then, in the third step, the team reports on the outcome of the consultation to the referring unit, in order to help reorient their action plan, while using the specific case to raise broader issues around cultural dynamics and social inequalities in health and social care.

In the first step described above, the team explains the CCC's theoretical framework and methodology, highlighting the differences from the approach that is normally used in health and social care settings in Italy for addressing 'cultural' issues: relying on cultural and linguistic mediation. Such an approach is generally rooted in the highly problematic idea that cultural factors are relevant only when dealing with foreigners, while bio-medical knowledge is culture-free. Moreover, the rationale behind cultural and linguistic mediation is the questionable assumption that people coming from the same geographical area have the same culture.

The CCC operates with an alternative vision, asserting that cultural dynamics intersect all aspects of social life, including biomedical knowledge and health and social care services, and that focusing on the cultural aspects of the illness experience is problematic unless socioeconomic forces are taken equally into consideration (Farmer, 2003). In fact, we cannot ignore that the suffering of migrants is often deeply tied to the personal em-bodiment of normative, social, and economic processes of marginalization (Farmer, 1999; Fassin, 2001a, 2001b; Krieger, 2005; Ticktin, 2011). Following this vision, the CCC's multidisciplinary team works to address both the symbolic dimensions involved as well as the social processes that contribute to producing suffering by limiting access to fundamental resources.

Throughout the consultation process, the CCC adopts an empiric and dynamic view of culture: not just in terms of 'something we have' as members of a certain group or community, but also in terms of 'something we make' in the intersubjective process of interacting with others. From this theo-retical standpoint, CCC's intervention is not aimed at promoting patients' compliance, but rather at producing data in the very interaction with all the involved actors, including the patient as well as the referring professionals.

In biomedical debates, and in the use of cultural and linguistic mediation, one hears a common refrain of 'taking care of the patient's perspective', as if this was pre-existing and ready to be shared. What happens when the patient does not have a perspective to be taken care of? How can such a situation come about?

The anthropological contribution to CCC consultation activities can be appreciated in its focus on culture as a process rooted in practices, accord-ing to which personal experience is appreciated as the lived dimension of cultural processes. Within this approach, personal crisis, whether related to illness or to other dimensions of one's existence, is seen as capable of projecting the person into a context in which everyday meanings are at risk. What is usually taken for granted, in the processual flow of our daily existence, ceases to allow a 'naturalized' being in the world, and thus creates a need to reflexively engage in a (new) meaning-making process.[2]

---

2   Byron Good (1994) talked about such a process in terms of the un-making of the lifeworld; Ernesto De Martino (1958) in terms of the crisis of presence; Linda Garro (1992) in terms of an ontological assault.

Within this framework, the CCC adopts a narrative approach not only to investigate social practices in cultural terms, but as a cultural practice in itself, to support the patient in exploring his/her own ideas and beliefs. The aim is helping people to discern and clarify their needs. Following Sally Gadow (1980), and Annemarie Mol (2008) more recently, the CCC chooses the right to meaning as the starting point: rather than aiming to involve patients in making an informed choice on a proposed therapeutic plan, the CCC works to explicitly engage them in first producing the meaning of their situation. This is the step from which the possibility of making a choice can emerge. The CCC has found that involving the patient in the production of the meaning of his/her situation can transform the very experience of what is happening.

Working on the right to meaning has proven to be productive, but certainly not sufficient, unless other rights can be claimed and met at the same time. We can thus summarize the process using the following expression: 'from narrative to empowerment'. On the one hand, a narrative approach risks being ineffective, unless the comprehension it produces gives rise to some kind of empowerment. On the other hand, if we don't involve patients in the meaning-making process, and we assume we know what is in their best interest, we risk promoting forms of action that are not rooted in their local moral world. Both approaches are problematic if divided from one another.

In the following discussion of specific cases, I argue that their resolution was not so much the result of a successful mediation and negotiation between different perspectives, but rather stemmed from a process that transformed experience, in other words, subjectivity, by activating the social resources required for agency to be played out. In this sense, the CCC works both to promote patients' participation and to foster institutional reflexivity, in order to help the staff themselves to become agents of transformation.

The case of Ghalia: From the right to meaning to empowerment

Ghalia was a woman in her mid-40s who came to Italy from Morocco to join her husband, with whom she has three children, aged fifteen, five, and four. The CCC began to work on her case in April 2011, after being activated by the social service unit that was following the entire family group. The unit was requesting a psychiatric evaluation for the woman, as the staff thought she was affected by some form of mental health disorder. We explained to the unit that our role was not that of making a diagnosis but rather helping the social service unit to deal with the case.

The husband had divorced her as he felt she was behaving in a strange way, including believing in the evil eye and bewitching, and her relationship with the children had deteriorated as she had stopped taking care of them. During a fight between the parents the police had to intervene and eventually the husband paid rent for a new house in which Ghalia went to live with the two younger children, while the oldest opted to stay with the father. After a while, things fell apart as Ghalia did not use the money her husband gave her to pay the rent, instead flying to Morocco, where she took her case to a tribunal in order to obtain adequate economic support from her former husband. She showed herself to be assertive and capable of sensibly planning her actions.

When she returned to Italy, though, she could not go back to her house, as the owner had reported her to the social service unit for not paying the rent. Ghalia was then taken into custody by the service and offered a place in a house for women in need. In the house, where she lived with other women and social service staff, her behaviour was described as being even stranger than before (she feared specific colours, she did not want to wash herself and her children, she was very aggressive with social workers and educators, etc.), so much so that her competence as a mother was questioned and the suggestion was made to refer the children to juvenile court.

During the consultation process Ghalia was initially confused and did not understand what she was supposed to say and do. During several encounters we invited her to tell us her story and she slowly came to articulate her ideas, expressing hostile feelings towards the social service unit for having an authoritative attitude, and most of all for using her children as a way to blackmail her, saying: 'If you do not comply with this and that, the court will take your children away.' The social service unit, on the other hand, insisted that she did not seem capable of caring for her children's needs, and looked for a psychiatric explanation for her 'strange' behaviour.

The consultation with Ghalia made it clear that her negative feelings towards her husband and his family had taken the cultural form of bewitchment, and that her refusal to wash herself and the children was a way of rejecting her role as wife and mother under the circumstances in which she was living while separated from her husband. Moreover, the arranged marriage she had been forced into was never fully accepted by her, as it meant abandoning her university studies in Morocco in order to join the husband in Italy, where he had a permanent position in a factory. She perceived her migrant situation as a diminishment of her social status, lacking a proper social network and support. Throughout the consultation meetings, Ghalia started to make up her mind; slowly coming to terms with the divorce, she found she felt trapped anyway, as she did not see herself in a socially legitimated and appreciated role. She was no longer a wife, she certainly did not want to go back to Morocco, and she had no friends or relatives in Italy. In light of these factors, she began to consider her role as a mother as the only one that could give sense to her present life. It was a role, though, that she had to reinvent from scratch.

This case highlights how the CCC uses ethnography: the anthropologists involved intentionally adopted an approach aimed at engaging Ghalia in the co-construction of meaning. The consultation as ethnography is not only a data-collecting process used to investigate social practices in cultural terms, but rather a cultural practice that enables people to produce a perspective on their experience. Such a re-positioning of Ghalia, centred on her intention to reframe her social role as mother, transformed the situation. In fact, as part of the process that reshaped the meanings of the situation, the attitude of the social service unit also came to a change: as a different line of reasoning emerged, they agreed to help Ghalia to find a house and a job that could increase her autonomy. In the meantime, what they perceived as 'strange' in her behaviour was no longer framed in the terms of a psychiatric condition.

What the social service unit initially expected from us was a cultural (or, maybe, culturalist) analysis of the case in order to proceed with a psychiatric diagnosis, thus shifting to others the responsibility of taking care of a problematic relationship, and allowing for the referral of the children to juvenile court. The main challenge for them was to manage such a complex case without having the resources they felt they needed. In this respect, the reshaping of healthcare and welfare—including market-oriented reforms, budget cuts, and privatization—has increased the fragmentation of services and reduced their ability to mobilize and access resources.

During the process of consultation, the attitude of those involved changed dramatically. Ghalia became increasingly assertive and less elusive, clearer about herself and her needs, and more determined to achieve her goals: a place to stay alone with her children, a peaceful relationship with her former husband in order to re-establish a connection with her oldest son, and a job. The social service unit was relieved from shouldering the burden of a case for which the staff felt inadequate and unprepared. What made the difference was the participation of all the actors involved in defining the nature of the reality at stake, which created the feeling of being all on the same side. In this way, change was brought about by those primarily—and institutionally—involved, and not by the CCC team. It was not sharing information that led to a different course of action, but rather participating in the production of meaning that transformed people's experience and attitudes.

The case of Nabil: Inhabiting institutional contradictions

Nabil, in his early 30s, also came from Morocco, and was born with a slight cognitive impairment. After arriving in Italy with his mother and siblings to join his father, in 2000, he was taken to the local mental health unit and diagnosed as oligophrenic and schizophrenic. Following Nabil's diagnosis, the family obtained social subsidies from the municipality: a free house and support from the social services for finding a job for Nabil and promoting his social inclusion. Nabil's father mentioned during the consultation that his son had had motor and linguistic problems since birth, and that he experienced outbursts of anger. In the father's understanding, due to Nabil's language problems, anger and crying were his way of communicating.

The problems began when Nabil had a serious fight at work: while he was cleaning a space in the factory where he was employed, a worker walked intentionally on the wet floor he had cleaned and insulted Nabil with racist terms. Nabil lost his temper and assaulted him with a screwdriver. After this episode Nabil lost his job and stayed at home, until his father asked again the social service unit to help him find a new contract. After a while, Nabil started working as a gardener with a social cooperative. He greatly enjoyed the new place, until he was reproached by an educator and lost his temper again. His employment was immediately suspended and the social service unit blamed Nabil for not taking the drugs that would help him keep his anger under control. Because of his lack of compliance with the prescribed treatment, he was judged unreliable. The situation was further complicated by the fact that Nabil did not want his family to know why he had lost the second job, creating even more tensions between him and his father.

During the consultation, Nabil was furious with his father and with the social service unit, and accused the CCC team of being yet another form of oppression. After providing a space in which he was asked to reflect on his wishes and needs, he slowly came to realize that he wanted some kind of independence from his family (and their control). He wanted to go back to work and socialize with other people; this emerged as a problematic issue, as Nabil tended to get along with other Moroccans 'who sell dope and waste time in the streets', as his father put it. However, his diagnosis made it impossible for him to apply for a job without the support of the social service unit, which was in turn tied to his compliance with treatment. Nabil felt trapped in the role of the sick person by his family's poor economic condition, as his disability was the only ground on which they could claim housing benefits, and he felt oppressed by the social service unit that considered him a child, unreliable and needing care.

Throughout the consultation a new picture emerged: despite his cognitive impairment, Nabil demonstrated more and more confidence in asserting his wishes, showing considerable capacity for autonomous judgement. He emphasized how fast he was learning Italian (despite the diagnosis describing him as very limited in communication skills), and characterized his anger as a reasonable—though excessive—reaction to offences and/or patronizing attitudes that he found unacceptable and racist. The social worker in charge of his case confirmed that he was indeed very good at adapting to new working contexts and that he easily made friends. All these elements suggested the need to re-evaluate Nabil's clinical situation: the doctor who had made the diagnosis of oligophrenia and schizophrenia was then involved in the consultation and agreed to reassess the case.

At this point, though, the CCC team faced a profound contradiction: the anthropological understanding of the social circumstances within which Nabil's story had unfolded suggested the need to reframe his condition in more social rather than medical terms; yet being labelled as disabled was the (only) means through which his family could access essential support. Eventually, Nabil himself found the solution: he was ready to adopt (and adapt to) the role of 'disabled' if this could increase his independence, demonstrating once again his ability to negotiate the terms of his existence. He agreed to take depot medications, thus reassuring the services that he would not skip treatment. This would in turn allow him to get a job and gain his independence, while maintaining the disability status on which his family could keep claiming housing support. Presently Nabil has a job, takes part in several activities organized by the social service unit, and is a permanent member of a football team through which he gains social inclusion and personal satisfaction.

Open questions as a way of concluding

How was it that, in both cases, Ghalia and Nabil managed to slowly come to discern and better understand their desires and needs? How did this process ease the stress that social and healthcare services were experiencing in dealing with patients described as highly problematic? In both cases, cultural and linguistic mediators had been called for help, without finding an effective way to manage the situation.

The consultation process revealed that social and healthcare services are structurally framed in a way that impedes people's participation in producing a meaning of themselves and their situation. In fact, professionals tend to define people's problems in the terms of the service they can provide—they frame the diagnosis according to the treatment they can offer. It is not a personal or moral problem related to the good or bad intention of the individual worker, rather a structural and epistemological issue related to the social organization of welfare services and to the forms of knowledge that are socially legitimated within them.

By limiting people's participation in the production of meaning of their own situation, professionals are unintentionally contributing to their own ineffectiveness. In contrast, by fostering an intersubjective view of culture as a dynamic process that originates from the practical engagement of all involved actors, the CCC not only stayed away from an essentialized view of cultural differences, but also empowered the social service unit by exposing the cultural dimensions embedded in any care relationship, enabling the staff to become agents of change.

In both cases, the third step of the consultation process focused on some broader issues, starting from that of communication, given the role it plays in the legal framework within which social and healthcare services work. In fact, for Ghalia as well as for Nabil, communicating information did not lead to informed choice and action. On the contrary, action emerged only after a meaning-making process was triggered. Through creating the conditions for their participation in such a process, their experience emerged as transformed.

In order to support and sustain such a transformation, it was necessary to act also on the socioeconomic context where the disease had arisen. While exposing culture as an intersubjective process of meaning production through which we give sense to reality and create our experience of it, the CCC's approach also highlights how such a step is only the basis for identifying at what level action must be undertaken. In other words: understanding does not necessarily solve the problem, action must follow.

I propose we consider efficacy in terms of transformation: if reductionism is the very ground for biomedical efficacy by creating the condition for a technical intervention capable of transforming anatomical and physiological aspects of individual (bio)existence, then, likewise, granting patients the right to meaning can produce a transformation of their experience, which in turn must be sustained through action upon the social circumstances of their existence. In a nutshell, by promoting the right to meaning we come to understand how we may promote a different form of sociality, according to which the transformation of subjectivity can be carried out. By doing so we try to translate specific theoretical orientations into operational tools geared towards human and institutional capacity building, to counteract the fragmentation of experience produced by the organization of welfare services into separate compartments, culturally framed according to biological, psychological, or social distinctions.

In the participatory action-research framework adopted by the CCC, health and social care services must be involved in order to create the premises for them to effectively address the problems they face. Trapped in forms of knowledge and organizations rooted in a hegemonic cultural understandings and institutional protocols, professionals clearly express their need for increased institutional reflexivity in order to rethink their own role within those institutions. Such an approach implies the direct involvement of the anthropologist with the reality s/he is working in; it could not be otherwise, as we all well know as ethnographers. Such an involvement, though, is not without consequences and contradictions, as seen in the case of Nabil, in which the possibility of demedicalizing his condition did not work in his own and his family's best interest. Who is entitled to define what the best interest of a person is? How do we come to label a certain action as agentive? In these two cases, the value of a specific action or interpretation clearly depended on the social consequences it produced in the patient's world, mediated in turn by his/her position in the broader (yet local) social context.

Thus we come to appreciate the need to analyse the tensions and relationships existing between socially positioned *forms of life* and *bare life,* seen as a product of an institutional assemblage of actors, knowledge, and practices. Access to essential support is granted by the institutional production of specific kinds of subjectivity (good nurturing mother, disabled person) that, however, do not cancel out people's agency. In fact, agency can be appreciated in terms of the possibility to critically engage the processes of one's own construction/constriction, thus producing a transformation of one's own existence.

The CCC had to face another contradiction: accessing healthcare and social services with the mandate of working on the relationship with migrants, given the public and institutional understanding of 'culture' as being relevant only when dealing with foreigners (particularly if coming from the Global South). In the long run, the CCC aims to contribute to social and healthcare services that are based on social equity and cultural sensitivity, no matter where the patient comes from. However, for the time being administrators and decision makers are ready to address these issues exclusively in the field of migration. It was within this context that the CCC project was accepted and introduced in the provincial welfare plan, because it was perceived as a tool to help improve patients' compliance with the services' prescriptions. By accepting such a contradiction, though, the CCC produced a different outcome: reorienting the whole action plan of the involved services.

The issue of public anthropology is then a complex one, which goes well beyond normative guidelines to imply a direct engagement in an ever-changing reality that requires an ethical standpoint based on questions rather than final answers. Public anthropology has the potential to have a social and institutional impact through exploring and inhabiting the tensions and contradictions existing between *bare life* and *forms of life*, and by translating its theoretical devices into operational strategies that combine symbolic analysis with social engagement. In doing so, anthropologists certainly need to build alliances with social and healthcare professionals, not just in terms of increasing the efficacy and efficiency of existing services, but also by interjecting their needs and creating the conditions for their participation in a different framework of reflection and action, one that is capable of making their best interests compatible with those of their patients.

For doing so, we must move towards a multidisciplinary and multimethod approach, framing health and social care as processes that transform experience by acting on the reconfiguration of the symbolic and social circumstances within which persons can emerge as subjects—as socially recognized and legitimate actors. Health is certainly a cultural construct, but it must be socially generated through an engagement that—while not devoid of contradictions—calls for a processual reflexivity based on shared responsibility in defining what is transformative and agentive, for whom, and according to what social circumstances.

References

Agamben, G. (1998). *Homo sacer*. Stanford: Stanford University Press.

Agamben, G. (2005). *State of exception*. Chicago: University of Chicago Press.

Butler, J. (1997). *The psychic life of power: Theories in subjection*. Stanford: Stanford University Press.

Comaroff, J. (2006). Oltre la politica della nuda vita: L'AIDS e l'ordine neoliberista. In I. Quaranta, ed., *Annuario di antropologia. Vol. 8: Sofferenza sociale*. Rome: Meltemi.

De Martino, E. (1958). *Morte e pianto ritual: Dal lamento funebre antico al pianto di Maria*. Turin: Boringhieri.

Farmer, P. (1999). *Infections and inequalities: The modern plagues*. Berkeley: University of California Press.

Farmer, P. (2003). *Pathologies of power: Health, human rights, and the new war on the poor*. Berkeley: University of California Press.

Fassin, D. (2000). Entre politiques du vivant et politiques de la vie: Pour une anthropologie de la santé. *Anthropologie et sociétés, 24*(1), 95–116.

Fassin, D. (2001a). The biopolitics of otherness. *Anthropology Today, 17*(1), 3–7.

Fassin, D. (2001b). Culturalism as ideology. In C.M. Obermeyer, ed., *Cultural perspectives on reproductive health* (pp. 300–317). Oxford: Oxford University Press.

Fassin, D. (2010). *La Raison Humanitaire: Une histoire morale du temps present.* Paris: Gallimard/Seuil.

Fassin, D., and Pandolfi, M., eds. (2010). *Contemporary states of emergency.* New York: Zone.

Gadow, S. (1980). Existential advocacy: Philosophical foundation of nursing. In S.F. Spiker and S. Gadow, eds., *Nursing: Images and ideas* (pp. 79–101). New York: Springer.

Garro, L. (1992). Chronic illness and the construction of narratives. In M.-J. Del Vecchio Good, P. Brodwin, B. Good, and A. Kleinman, eds., *Pain as human experience: An anthropological perspective* (pp. 100–137). Berkeley: University of California Press.

Good, B. (1994). *Medicine, rationality and experience.* Cambridge: Cambridge University Press.

Krieger, N., ed. (2005). *Embodying inequality: Epidemiologic perspectives.* Amityville: Baywood.

Mol, A.M. (2008). *The logic of care: Health and the problem of patient choice.* London: Routledge.

Moore, H. (2007). *The subject of anthropology: Gender, symbolism and psychoanalysis.* Cambridge: Polity Press.

Nguyen, V.-K. (2005). Antiretroviral globalism, biopolitics, and therapeutic citizenship. In A. Ong and S. Collier, eds., *Global assemblages: Technology, politics, and ethics as anthropological problems* (pp. 124–144). Malden: Blackwell.

Nguyen, V.-K. (2006). Attivismo, farmaci anti-retrovirali e riplasmazione del sé come forme di cittadinanza biopolitica. In I. Quaranta, ed., *Annuario di antropologia. Vol. 8: Sofferenza sociale.* Rome: Meltemi.

Ong, A. (2003). *Buddha is hiding: Refugees, citizenship, the new America.* Berkeley: University of California Press.

Ortner, S. (2006). *Anthropology and social theory: Culture, power, and the acting subject.* Durham: Duke University Press.

Petryna, A. (2002). *Life exposed: Biological citizens after Chernobyl.* Princeton: Princeton University Press.

Rose, N., and Novas, C. (2005). Biological citizenship. In A. Ong and S. Collier, eds., *Global assemblages: Technology, politics, and ethics as anthropological problems* (pp. 439–463). Malden: Blackwell.

Ticktin, M. (2011). *Casualties of care: Immigration and the politics of humanitarianism in France.* Berkeley: University of California Press.

Werbner, R. (2002). Postcolonial subjectivities: The personal, the political and the moral. In R. Werbner, ed., *Postcolonial subjectivities in Africa* (pp. 1–21). London: Zed Books.

Whyte, S.R. (2009). Health identities and subjectivities: The ethnographic challenge. *Medical Anthropology Quarterly, 23*(1), 6–15.

Part III
NEW SOCIALITIES AND SUBJECTIVITIES IN CARE

7   Muslim migrants in Montreal and perinatal care

Challenging moralities and local norms

Sylvie Fortin and Josiane Le Gall

Stemming from multisited research on Muslim migrants in Montreal and perinatal care,[1] this paper centres on the local and transnational socialities in regards to perinatal knowledge as well as how these socialities and knowledge-sharing practices become actors in the local clinical encounter. We address these two themes within a pluralistic setting, where health services (whether community or tertiary) seek to adjust to local demographic changes (31% of Montrealers are born outside of Canada (Statistics Canada, 2007)).[2] For more than a decade, Muslim countries have been among the leading home countries of Montreal's migrants, making Islam (mostly Sunnite) the second religion in Quebec, after Catholicism.

Families of all backgrounds share perinatal knowledge that is passed on from one generation to the next (Cresson and Mebtoul, 2010). Yet, this knowledge changes over time and place (Hjelm et al., 2009; Grewal et al., 2008; Boyacioglu and Türkmen, 2008; Yount, 2007). How it is met within clinical encounters with Muslim migrants gives rise to a number of questions, particularly in regards to gender roles, family dynamics, and decision-making processes related to healthcare issues (Ny et al., 2007, 2008; Pels, 2000; Fortin and Le Gall, 2012; Fortin, 2013b).

In this contribution, we discuss socialities in the context of migration, with special attention to the changing role of fathers and how these socialities are involved in the clinical encounter. We see that expert knowledge

1   The pluridisciplinary research team that led this study funded by the Canadian Research Health Institutes (2007– 2012) was composed of S. Fortin, J. Le Gall, G. Bibeau (anthropologists); A. Payot, F. Audibert (clinicians); F. Carnevale and A. Gagnon (nurses); and many research assistants: M. Bélanger and S. Maynard (successively team coordinators); R. SiAllouch, M. Rietmann, C. Thériault, and É. Fréchette Audy; as well as G. Désilet, L. Benhadjoudja, A. Adouane, A. Détole, and J. Letarte.

2   Montreal's historical migrant diversity gives rise to a dynamic plural locality. This cosmopolitan metropolis welcomes from 40,000 to 50,000 migrants per year from more than a hundred different countries (Gouvernement du Québec, 2013).

is rarely questioned, and examine how perceived gender relationships and inequalities shape clinical discourses and practices, despite (or due to) a greater involvement of the father in the perinatal sphere. In examining the varied habitus of the caregiver/patient interaction, we make sense of the values, norms, and practices that emerge and how they shape subjectivities.[3] We conclude by situating these socialities and subjectivities within a broader context and noting how the contrasting different logics help us understand our future socialities.

Methodology

The main goal of the study was to analyse the encounter between Muslim families and healthcare providers (HCPs), paying particular attention to the negotiation of knowledge, norms, and values as well as familial and professional practices. Observations were carried out in Montreal, in the obstetrics and neonatal wards of two university tertiary paediatric hospitals, one university general hospital, as well as during perinatal activities in several front-line community healthcare establishments (prenatal group meetings, breastfeeding clinics, programmes for low-income pregnant women, postnatal visits at home).[4] Over a two-year period, we repeatedly attended unit meetings, observed daily practices of the obstetrical and neonatal wards, shadowed community nurses on their home visits (all mothers in Quebec are seen at home a few days following childbirth), and attended perinatal activities.

Findings were also collected from semi-structured interviews with 54 HCPs (15 hospital physicians, 12 hospital and 20 community nurses and 7 other professionals (psychologist, nutritionist, social worker) in the community or hospital setting), and 95 Muslim mothers recruited in these

3   There are multiple definitions of subjectivity. It is a rich and complex notion that embraces 'continuity and diversity of personhood' while taking into account the different processes that participate in its making (Biehl et al., 2007, p. 1). For anthropologists, subjectivities are 'landscapes of explosions', 'noise', and 'disconnects and dissociations' mixed with 'reason' and 'rationalizations', all of which have sociopolitical dimensions (Fisher, 2007, p. 424). For our part, we understand it to be the delicate relationship between the construct and the perception, an approach that combines in the same instant experience and background; structure, agency and interaction; the individual; and his/her path in relation to political, economic, and historical conditions in which this course occurs.

4   Our study was approved by the ethics review board of all participating institutions.

institutions, of which 20 became case studies.[5] We met repeatedly with the latter (a mean of five encounters per case) during pregnancy and in the first months of motherhood, as well as with their spouse and any other household figure (friend or family member) present in the home, or in the community activity space or hospital clinic at the time of our study. The interviews with the HCPs were all conducted in French (Quebec being a French-speaking province in all public affairs). The interviews with the mothers were conducted in French or in English and secondarily in Arabic or another language (with a translator), upon the mother's choice.

The majority of the women interviewed were from North Africa (63%), mainly Morocco and Algeria, which are among the top countries of origin of the recent immigrant population in Quebec, the others being mostly from South Asia/Indian subcontinent (15%) and the Middle East (14%). Most of these mothers (80%) had been in Montreal for less then five years (and in fact, 55% had been in Montreal less than two years). Many of these women (50%) and their spouses (67%) had a university degree and spoke French on a daily basis (68%). They nevertheless encountered numerous difficulties entering the mainstream workforce. The majority affirmed being 'practicing believers' (of Islam).

As for the HCP, most (76%, 41/54) were non-migrants (Canadian born of French descent) while the others came from an array of localities (European, Middle Eastern, North African, Asian, or Caribbean). While the vast majority were of Catholic faith (83%, 45/54), only a few (29%, 13/45) affirmed being 'practicing or moderate practitioners' of their religion. With the exception of one HCP, those of Muslim, Jewish, or Buddhist faith were all 'practicing or moderate practitioners'.

Local and transnational socialities in regards to perinatal knowledge

The perinatal period, particularly for primiparous women, can be quite a 'test' in the context of migration. Some of the daily challenges include accessing and understanding the local healthcare system, sharing knowledge, and gaining regular everyday support. The care of other children is an

---

5   Case studies included a formal interview (as with all respondents) and several informal exchanges with the mother, her spouse, and any other family member or friend present, as well as observations of clinical encounters, community activities, and home dynamics.

additional challenge for multiparous women who, in their places of origin, often benefitted from significant support at this stage of life.

In Montreal, 90 out of 95 mothers interviewed lived in 'nuclear' families.[6] While more than half of the mothers encountered (52%) had at least one family member in Montreal (often siblings close or far), the support provided by extended family at the time of birth was found to be limited (only 33% had experienced this).[7] Beyond the family, local friendships (often of the same ethnic background) or neighbours nearby are also a source of support and knowledge (for 71% of mothers interviewed) with regard to the care of the newborn in the broader respect of available public services (information or accompaniment), providing useful accessories for the perinatal period or emotional and material support (cooking, dishes), etc. One woman told us:

> They come over, they talk to me on the phone all the time. And yes, they try to make me laugh. [...] Because they know, they have experience. They don't stop calling. They come [...] and bring Algerian dishes. I don't know these people [Algerian women she encountered at the park or whose kids know each other]. There was even one woman who brought me everything I needed—the baby bath, [...] clothes, things, many things. (Samia, Algeria, multiparous, in Montreal for less than two years)

While support from the extended family in Montreal is scarce, many mothers seek advice from family members living in the country of origin, especially from the mother (recently or about to become grandmother). Virtual support (via telephone, Internet), on a quasi-daily basis, will be given in response to requests for advice on pregnancy and mothering, and knowledge about food, nutrition, and care of the newborn. During periods of 'lying in', however, a third of the women (all from the Maghreb) benefitted from the presence of a mother or stepmother who travelled from the homeland to support them. As described by a new 'grandmother' from Morocco: 'I cooked, did laundry, washed the dishes, I took care of the newborn. [...] I slept with her for three days in the hospital.' The women interviewed unambiguously demonstrated the importance of this virtual sociality during pivotal moments of the perinatal period. Important decisions that

6   For the other four (of Indian, Pakistani, or Afghan origin), they lived within a more extended grouping of the husband's family (in-laws and/or siblings of the husband).

7   In the home localities, the involvement of the family follows a typically vertical structure of support, with the mother (or stepmother) helping the daughter (or daughter-in-law), and more rarely a horizontal pattern (intragenerational support).

can affect a pregnancy (at risk), the intention (or not) to do a screening test (such as amniocentesis), the possibility of an abortion in the case of a negative diagnosis or prognosis or anything that falls within neonatology (and the many decisions surrounding different treatments or withdrawal from treatment)—in short, all these situations give rise to a search for advice in response to complex issues for which the family or the mother of the respondent is widely sought. In a similar fashion, if the mother or mother-in-law is visiting Montreal (notably for the 'lying-in' period (*les relevailles*)), she will take an active part in the decision-making that affects the couple. Spiritual guides might also be solicited to help with decision-making during these 'pivotal' moments. As such, the relationship with religion is often inseparable from the decisions that will impact perinatal life and death. In effect, it becomes an integral part of sociality, whether it be local or transnational. At the same time, the quest for less-invested knowledge is commonly channelled through the Internet and accessible literature. As Maisah, from Pakistan states:

> One thing we noticed in Pakistan is that the information only comes from parental or close peers who have gone through the experience. Here, I guess it's more like, you know, website, books and everything. [...] So I was just like buying books and we were just reading and that's, so we kind of got it from both ways. (Maisah, Pakistan, multiparous, in Montreal for less than two years)

Women also choose what knowledge is best:

> You know common sense, at the end common sense. Yeah I listen to my mother but I listen to the doctor too and I read a lot. So if you read a lot, and because they gave me a lot things to read, I was always searching on the Net for definitions of what to do, what not to do. So I was ready, if my mother gives me advice, I will like just know by common sense that this is right. (Zeina, Lebanon, mutliparous, in Montreal for less than two years)

Family dynamics and gender roles in the making

Mothers are likely to remember the quality of support present in the locality of origin compared to life in the context of migration:

> The difference is that here [in Montreal], several times I've thought, I've wondered: Is it a good decision to have a baby? Who will help me? Who

will take care of me? In Morocco, I didn't worry about that, I didn't ask myself these questions because I had my family by my side. [For my first pregnancy in Morocco] they helped me enormously, everyone, my sisters, my mother. They took care of me, they prepared the food. Up until the third month after the birth, I was still at my mother's. (Nora, Morocco, multiparous, in Montreal for two years)

Although family presence is often longed for, some women point to the advantages of living at an extended family distance:

Maybe, I guess it's nice to have your family around, you know, and your friends as well [in the homeland]. But here, maybe I was more relaxed because it was more quiet for me. Like, I wake up whenever I want with my baby and I sleep whenever I want, you know. Each place has its advantages and disadvantages. Back in Saudi Arabia, everyone wants to see the baby and everyone wants to come to visit and it will be very busy for us. But at the same time, I will have more help. But here I think, he's a very quiet baby. You know? He just wakes up, feeds, has his diaper changed, and sleeps. And now I'm not working. I'll start working in July. My baby will go to the day care at the same time. So, yeah, it's comfortable and it's quiet. Like we love to be in a quiet place, you know, yeah. (Sara, Saudi Arabia, multiparous, in Montreal for less than two years)

In the same way, a Turkish mother (primiparous, in Montreal for five years) shares with us her mixed feelings in regards to her in-laws. Since the birth of her daughter, her in-laws have been living with her, helping out. She considers all this help too much and expresses the desire to see them live more at a distance. Two weeks after childbirth, she has yet to change a diaper. At the same time she says she feels guilty after having such thoughts, knowing that the in-laws will miss their granddaughter once they are back in Turkey in a few months' time. But could they help out more with the house chores and less with the baby? As a mother, she appears to feel left aside and to fear the baby's bonding with her mother-in-law. Abir similarly recalled her 'lying-in' period in Lebanon, telling us that she felt like the message was 'the baby is no longer yours' (Abir, primiparous, in Montreal for one year).

In other words, the 'nuclearization' of the perinatal period is not only a sombre process. Some women experience a reconfiguration of roles and responsibilities, an easing of social expectations associated with the birth of a child, or even greater autonomy.

> Yes, at my place, my mother came over [from Algeria]. There were too many visitors. It was a bit tiring, especially for my mother—she took care of the baby and of the visitors. You don't have any private time with your husband. [...] That's why I liked it here. We enjoyed the arrival of the baby with [our] family. Father and children, that's all. (Hezora, Algeria, multiparous, in Montreal for two years)

Zeina, a Lebanese mother (primiparous, in Montreal for less than two years), also mentioned how her pregnancy away from home and the independence she developed throughout her maternity helped her to become autonomous. Had she been in Lebanon, she said, she would have been cared for by her family (her mother and mother-in-law, in particular) and she would not have learned to care for her child.

Migration (and the perinatal period) also favours change in the couple and family dynamics: the new father becomes an actor in the foreground.[8] A large percentage (67%) of the mothers mentioned the increased participation of the husband, who accompanied them to and interpreted at medical appointments, neonatal care, or during delivery, as well as assisting in everyday household and family tasks (Fortin and Le Gall, 2012). Whether running errands, preparing meals, or taking care of older children, fathers occupy a new ground within the family:

> After the birth, he was very sincerely involved. Very present—well, he didn't really have any other choice. Who will help me? He didn't have a choice. [...] There is no one here with me, there is just him, so he is obligated. And especially for men at home, it's not easy for them to get involved, they are spoiled, they do nothing. No, they do nothing, it's just the woman. [...] I'm talking about home, tradition is like that. For the men, it's just work outside the home. But here they are forced to [help] [...], it's the culture. But [in my home country] we don't need them, really. There is the mother, the sisters, there is all of that so [husbands] don't do anything. It's just a psychological support or you know, moral support. Otherwise, for the house, [we are well] surrounded: you have your mother, you have your sister, your friends. (Nadine, Morocco, primiparous, in Montreal for five years)

---

8   Migration can indeed result in an increase of paternal involvement due to the diminished family network and the greater availability of men (limited social network, lack of work). See also Le Gall and Cassan (2010) on this topic.

As a Mauritanian husband (multiparous spouse in Montreal for five years) put it:

> Well, of course, it's very different from home and obviously if it would have happened there, I would have been less involved because there are plenty of things that—it's ok, it will be done by the mother [of my spouse], the cooking, things like that. Here, well, I represent a little bit of everything. So it is a good experience and, as we said, it takes a lot of patience, a lot—but we must be ready.

The husbands' contribution will fade, however, with the arrival of a family member from the place of origin. The mother-in-law (or mother) often eclipses the father in the care of the newborn in terms of presence at the hospital. In the context of restrictive neonatal visits for example, it is not uncommon for fathers to transfer their visiting rights to a visiting family member.

Yet, for many fathers, accessing the obstetric ward is a novelty. In their home country this is often not possible, as the perinatal world is most often a woman's space. As Raghad's husband, Rashid, recalls in this exchange:

> Rashid: Yes, the difference is with the husband. The husband, they will not like his being involved in the pregnancy, like [the way it is] here. Here I'm involved, I feel I am involved a lot. In Libya I can't [do the same]. Well, I can't say 'no, I can't', but like, there is a custom, like how to deal with your wife—just call her mom or her sister or ask her to come and help her. And especially in the case room, or the delivery room, so maybe her mom or her sister will go with her inside.
>
> Interviewer: The husband usually doesn't go?
>
> Rashid: No, no, in Libya, no. And here like it's, it's good for me or for husbands to see how the wife gets tired from the delivery and the pregnancy. [...] So this is the good thing that gives the husband [knowledge] on how his wife gets tired and what pregnancy means exactly. (Rashid, Libya [husband of Raghad, primiparous], in Montreal for two years)

And from Tanisha's point of view:

> My husband, he was all the time with me. I think he did everything. He was a substitute for my family because I was worried that maybe I

would miss my mom during the delivery. So he was very, very good with me, emotionally, and he helped me in everything. Actually, he was with me in the, in the room where they're making the surgery, the C-section. Everything was good with him. (Tanisha, Syria, primiparous, in Montreal for less than two years)

In short, the here and the elsewhere meet virtually in the migratory context to offer emotional, informative, and moral support. Perinatal support may take the form of a mother or a mother-in-law visiting Montreal. If this is not to be, the husband often assumes a new role and demonstrates a level of participation often very different from his role in the place of origin. He takes an active part in various tasks in the household and is a more sustained presence in the healthcare institutions of Montreal.

How these socialities and knowledge-sharing practices become actors in the local clinical encounter

Knowledge and support

The large majority of the women interviewed consider HCPs to be (the most) significant source of information. Knowledge put forward by medical professionals, in the community as well as in the hospital setting, pose little or no problem with families accepting and adhering to this advice. This knowledge is perceived as a 'value-added' aspect of the local society. Biomedical knowledge is already esteemed key knowledge in the locality of origin although the conditions of public supply of medicine are often strongly criticized. The 'aura' surrounding biomedicine in North America plays favourably in the reception of different knowledge.

Expert knowledge is no less heterogeneous and sometimes even contradictory, depending on the practice settings (intra- and inter-institutional, hospital, and community care), the training environment (and time thereof), and the social paths. The clinical encounter is coloured just as is the negotiation of knowledge between experts and nonbelievers based on the healthcare settings. For example, nurses who visit new mothers in the context of an at-home, universal, postnatal care programme confirm that they gently modify their practice to manage each situation on case-by-case basis and adjust as necessary. To the extent that knowledge (and practices) do not harm the health of the mother or the baby and do not seem 'imposed' on them, the perspectives of the mothers and the extended family are valued. In discussing the risks associated with early pregnancy, a (community, non-migrant) nurse will say: 'They are told by their mother: "I did it myself, you are able to do it too."'

Overall, nurses are coping well with the various practices brought from the locality of origin, whether it be specific body treatments such as using clay, olive oil, or coconut oil on the baby's skin (for hydration), the shaving the newborn's hair (as an offering, or symbol of cleanliness), or how to swaddle the baby (to prevent bowleggedness). When a practice is perceived as problematic (by the HCP) such as excessively covering the baby (so that he falls asleep while being breastfed, doesn't drink enough, or sweats to the point of becoming lethargic), or giving the baby instant formula rather than breastfeeding, the nurse intercedes. They say that the 'security' of the baby is the key to this negotiation and insofar as it is not called into question, the sharing of knowledge is possible.

In addition, community nurses—given the nature of the care anchored in the locality have a near daily interaction with this population—recognize the valuable contribution of members of the extended family and the general importance of support in the migratory context. The nurses assert that they develop strategies of inclusion in their work with the mothers:

> The family can pose a problem at this level [excessive swaddling, early incorporation of infant formula], but for other things, the family is very supportive, like when the mother or mother-in-law is present, it is she who prepares meals for the woman. She will help her, giving the baby baths, give the woman massages so it is very helpful in this regard. It is concerning nursing advice that we sometimes have problems. (Community nurse, immigrant)

Otherness, evolving socialities, and challenging moralities

The clinical encounter or the patient/provider interaction is nonetheless a moment of negotiation, and may even be a clash, though less so in regards to medical knowledge (even when transnational medical advice is taken into account), but rather in the relational domain and in the decision-making process around birth, perinatal health, and death. Religious and cultural 'otherness', diversity of values, as well as evolving socialities (extended family members, gender relations, parental dynamics, and spiritual leaders) and social practices come into play, challenging moralities and local norms.

Religion

Hospital HCPs consider religion a problem or a barrier when families are making medical decisions that do not follow staff recommendations, particularly in end-of-life situations (that is, whether to terminate pregnancy because of major foetus anomalies or to limit medical assistance when newborns are severely impaired). The hospital practitioners also question the 'weight' of religion as it seems to limit the mother's autonomy, an important value within the healthcare system. Physicians speak of an invisible interlocutor during the clinical encounter. In their view, Muslim mothers rely most often on God when having to make important decisions. For example, religion may support the decision not to abort, to continue care, to refuse the use of contraceptives or different screening tests, including amniocentesis (despite the risk of trisomy 21, or Down syndrome). Doctors declare that Muslim women consider this decision as belonging to God, a position often endorsed by religious leaders who are consulted in this regard.[9] In some cases, religious leaders even become interlocutors in the clinical encounter, although exterior to the family, which is judged problematic by some doctors.

Otherwise, our data demonstrates how 'religious faith' can sometimes become an issue in the patient–provider relationship, particularly when religious or cultural markers are interpreted as signs of gender inequality. It is perceived that this 'religious faith'—in this case Muslim—is subordinate to gender relations (real or imagined) in the local society. Our study highlights how gender inequality (real or perceived)—so often associated with mothers who wear the veil, or with the couple's dynamics (if the woman is silent and the husband is the principal interlocutor)—is troublesome for many HCPs. In this regard, it is worth mentioning the influence of several factors (notably the migratory journey and religious affiliation) on the sensitivity of the staff to these questions (Le Gall and Xenocostas, 2011; Fortin, 2013a).

The father and gender inequalities

As mentioned earlier, the role of the father often evolves in the migratory context. Paradoxically, the behaviour of these fathers does not necessarily

---

9   Our work in other areas of the hospital with different populations brings us to the same conclusion: Deferring to God in the decision-making process is a shared practice among more 'orthodox' believers, whether Christian, Jewish, or Muslim (Fortin, 2013a, 2013b).

correspond to the conception of the paternal role put forward by local social policies and health facilities, leading to frustration among fathers and HCPs alike (Le Gall et al., 2009; Ny et al., 2008). For some professionals, the father's role is perceived positively: they speak of 'support' and 'involvement', even if this involvement is gender differentiated (gendered tasks), saying things such as 'He takes to heart the whole family.' For others, often in the hospital setting, this role is discerned rather negatively and associated with gender inequalities (real or perceived): 'lack of involvement' in care and limited to positions of 'provision' or 'control'. These fathers are considered 'interventionist', 'claimants' who negotiate for the couple and 'speak for' their wives.

These gender dynamics become a real point of tension, a relational 'node' between the nurses, doctors (particularly women), and fathers. This tension extends to the mothers who consequently defend the involvement of their husbands in the household. As one HCP stated:

> I think what strikes me the most, what bothers me the most, is the role of the woman in that religion. The little power women have over their own decisions. That is the perception we have. From the very beginning, the first contact, they are always accompanied by their spouse. Often she doesn't respond to questions but rather her husband responds for her. If there are ever any decisions to make, it will be the husband and the imam. Maybe for us it troubles us to see that she does not control decisions that affect her. In effect, she has no autonomy for her person or pregnancy. So that's what confronts us the most in interacting with the Muslim population. I'm generalizing. They are not all like that, but there is a large percentage of Muslims like that and it really challenges us, it challenges our feminism, in our liberation to care for ourselves as women, it really gets us going. So we always try—it's stronger than us—I am convinced I am not alone in doing that [....], to impose a more direct communication with the woman. She is our patient, not the husband, not the imam, she is. (Obstetrician, non-immigrant)

From a different perspective, the male physicians say they see this dynamic at work, but that it doesn't affect them in the same way (idem for male nurses). For example, unlike the female staff, they associate more readily the interventionism of the father with a willingness to act as a 'linguistic mediator', or as a sort of 'buffer', and to relay information hoping to ease the situation for the wife rather than seeing it as a form of control over her. Overall, however, one impression dominates: the perception that the mother is not at the heart of decisions concerning herself or the child. Termination of pregnancy, birthing methods, and ending care for the newborn are rarely perceived by clinicians as decisions made or shared with the mother.

One mother, Radia (Algeria, multiparous, in Montreal for one year), to whom was announced a very grim prognosis for the baby she was carrying, chose, against the advice of the healthcare team, to continue the pregnancy. The entire team, in particular her obstetrician, was convinced that the mother did not show up for her medical appointment to abort the pregnancy under pressure from her husband. However, when we met Radia, she shared with us how she had wanted—against the will of her husband, but in agreement with her imam—to complete the pregnancy even if it should result in the death of the newborn. The husband had been upset by the choice of his wife, but accepted her quest for peace and her willingness to offer her (stillborn) child a burial following Muslim rites.

The perceptions of HCPs are, however, not fixed. An obstetrician admitted that what she first perceived as a lack of autonomy on the part of the mothers and as a lack of initiative (communication and decisions were mostly the domain of the husband) was later reinterpreted as a particular couple's dynamic at a specific stage in the trajectory of the couple and their migration, the husband having been an intermediary for the mother during hospitalization. Even if many of the women HCPs (non-migrants) involved with Radia's case were convinced of her submission to gender or religious domination, the neonatal physician (a migrant and a practicing Christian) read Radia's choices very differently:

> I find it difficult to live here in Quebec where late-term abortions are performed. [...] The child will die at birth so why not let him be born. We can give him love, palliative care, and he will die. [...] I feel like it is killing someone. [...] In Radia's case, I was relieved. I felt close to her and her family. [...] I shared their choice to go ahead with the pregnancy and cherished as they did, the importance of life. (Neonatal physician, migrant)

The extended family

The influence of the extended family (or of a member of the 'community') in the decision-making process is sometimes seen as positive, and other times as obstructing medical 'common sense'. Two examples illustrate this point:

> During treatment discontinuation in neonatology, a grandfather was helping the medical staff. Using verses from the Koran, he was explaining

to the parents that God, through the physicians, was somehow asking to take back the child. This discursive strategy made it possible to stop treatment whereas the prohibition to end a life is often at the heart of a disagreement between Muslim parents and care teams. (Observation notes, neonatal ward)

In another context, while the mother agreed (on medical advice) to a withdrawal of care, the father insisted on its continuation. Despite a grim and hopeless prognosis (the newborn was suffering from cerebral bleeding), the husband's family did not accept the discontinuation of care proposed by the team and exerted moral pressure on the father to make sure he did not retract from his position. Recognizing the treatment impasse, we asked an independent practitioner who engaged in discussions over several days, discussions inclusive of the parties involved. After this discussion period (some might say that it was too long to do so while the child was suffering, others will see this as the amount of time necessary to accept the end of a life…) we decided to end the treatment. (Observation notes, neonatal ward)

Conclusion

Our study documents social change in the making. Through the perinatal period, migrant women long for family and yet appreciate distance. Knowledge follows the family's path but is not the only means of gaining information. Many women choose what suits them best, whether that means following the advice of the family, religious leaders, or HCPs. As well, husband and wife relations evolve in the context of migration. Men feel concerned either by obligation (no other relative can support the expectant or new mother) or because they are invited to share an otherwise female domain. These different paths influence the clinical encounter where personal experiences, social milieu, community practices, and institutional cultures come into play. Moralities and norms evolve as knowledge is shared at different paces. Subjectivities are co-created, exposing a complex dialogue between individual experiences, wider social relations, and organizational issues. The healthcare paths of migrant Muslim women and their partners, the place of the extended family, or that of a spiritual guide seems for some to be awkward or unjust, and for others an important support. The dynamics specific to healthcare settings are not foreign to these divergent rationalities.

In community health services, diversity is expressed in everyday relationships, as the participating centres are located in the most plural, multi-ethnic settings in Montreal. Care delivery in the community is also based on proximity, as mothers encounter care on several occasions (through perinatal activities and at-home visits) in intimate settings. The sharing of knowledge is often the basis of the encounter between caregiver and patient; it is the result of subjectivities that fuel the relationship on a daily basis. Diversity is learned, discovered, negotiated. In contrast with the hospital context, though, community HCPs are less confronted with issues related to life and death where religious beliefs can come into conflict.

For the hospital, the often-critical interventions place the caregiver and the patient in very different positions where individual values can collide. The very organization of care, the multiplication of experts, the ever-present use of technological support—many elements are involved in the clinical encounter, not to mention the uncertainty of diagnosis and prognosis, and the relational uncertainty generated by this otherness (Fortin, 2013a). The clinical culture is also different: negotiation is a part of the learning process. In so doing, with a few exceptions, noncompliance with biomedical instructions (or suggested therapeutic guidance) is often explained by otherness, by different relational dynamics between couples, and by a connection to the collective and to religious belief that in turn become important actors in the clinical space. This noncompliance viewed through otherness hides an encounter of different rationalities (of different norms and values) constructed in very different habitus. The discontinuation of treatment, and its relation to life and death, doesn't have the same meaning for everyone. And if biomedicine sees treatment as a possible avenue because of a given diagnosis or prognosis, it may still be very different for the user, the mother, and the father.

Like Kaufman et al. (2006, 2011), we can relocate these gaps at the heart of differing subjectivities and temporalities, the one(s) from the clinical milieu and the one(s) from the patients and families. There are gaps based in the way we think about care, the values enshrined at the hearth of medical rationality, the weight of diagnosis and prognosis, and therefore what happens in the present. These concepts of future and present held by clinicians may be quite different for families. For the latter, biomedicine, with its often very wide therapeutic range and unprecedented technological support, fuels a hope that, along with one or the other conceptions of life, 'quality of life', and death, gives rise to the rationalities that may oppose those that have become standards in the clinical space. The ways of expressing these rationalities will in their turn match forms that reflect social, cultural, ethnic, and religious diversity present in any cosmopolitan environment.

Recognizing the gap or tensions between these rationales (Hacking, 1992), between community and tertiary hospital settings, between clinicians and families, is already recognizing that different rationalities coexist and that we gain by thinking of them as plural. Furthermore, thinking with religious diversity, in this context as well as social and cultural diversity—of the caregivers as well as of the cared for—is to think these rationalities as embedded not only in this patient/caregiver relation but in wider social rapports that cross any given society.

The 'religious fact' is defined differently according to the interlocutors and their personal orientation. The caregivers who are also 'believers', all faiths regrouped, are in general more receptive to the decisions of religious parents: the families' rationales resonate. For others, namely the caregivers of the local majority group, acknowledging religiously motivated decisions can sometimes (or often) be problematic and contribute to the shaping of otherness. In Quebec, this relation to religious belief cannot be fully understood outside of its recent history, notably the stranglehold that the Catholic Church had on (French-Canadian) society until the 1960s and the 'quiet Revolution' (Meintel and Fortin, 2002). The same is true concerning gender relations that particularly affect professionals from here and abroad. In so doing, the evolution of gender relations and relations to religion in the local society becomes the backdrop that we must grasp in order to better appreciate the importance these relations have in a caregiver–patient relationship.

Finally, the migratory path, the family structure, the forms of sociality, and their activation are all contexts that influence the clinical encounter, where norms and values crystallize and subjectivities get fuel. The different ways of relating to the 'religious fact' are constructed through time (colonial past, contemporary social structures), space (local, transnational), and, of course, depend on different religious currents and dogmas. To be interested in the clinical space allows us to better understand an ever-changing society, with all of the tensions that underline its vitality, a process 'in the making' instead of a context where everything is given and ordered (which in turn often reflects tighter borders between these different logics). Ultimately, following Zaman (2005) and Van der Geest and Finkler (2004), we reiterate the interest of thinking of the social space of the clinic as a 'capital of the mainland'.

References

Biehl, J., Good, B., and Kleinman, A. (2007). Introduction. In J. Biehl, B. Good, and A. Kleinman, eds., *Subjectivity* (pp. 1–23). Berkeley: University of California Press.

Boyacioglu, A.O., and Türkmen, A. (2008). Social and cultural dimensions of pregnancy and childbirth in eastern Turkey. *Culture, Health and Sexuality*, *10*(3), 277–285.

Cresson, G., and Mebtoul, M., eds. (2010). *Famille et santé*. Paris: Presses de l'EHESP.

Fisher, M.J. (2007). Epilogue: To live with what would otherwise be unendurable: Return(s) to subjectivities. In J. Biehl, B. Good, and A. Kleinman, eds., *Subjectivity* (pp. 423–446). Berkeley: University of California Press.

Fortin, S. (2013a). Conflits et reconnaissance dans l'espace social de la clinique: Les pratiques hospitalières en contexte pluraliste. *Anthropologie et sociétés*, *37*(3), 179–200.

Fortin, S. (2013b). Éthique(s) et prise de décision médicale en contexte de diversité. *Migrations Santé*, *146–147*, 17–51.

Fortin, S., and Le Gall, J. (2012). La parentalité et les processus migratoires. In F. De Montigny, A. Devault, and C. Gervais, eds., *La naissance de la famille: Accompagner les parents et les enfants en période périnatale* (pp. 178–196). Montréal: Chenelière Éducation.

Gouvernement du Québec (2013). *Migrations internationales et interprovinciales, Montréal et ensemble du Québec, 1996–1997, 2001–2002 et 2006–2007 à 2011–2012*. Retrieved from http://www.stat.gouv.qc.ca/statistiques/population-demographie/bilan2014.pdf.

Grewal, S.K., Bhagat, R., and Balneaves, L.G. (2008). Perinatal beliefs and practices of immigrant Punjabi women living in Canada. *Journal of Obstetric, Gynecologic, and Neonatal Nursing*, *37*(3), 290–300.

Hacking, I. (1992). The self-vindication of the laboratory sciences. In A. Pickering, ed., *Science as practice and culture* (pp. 26–62). Chicago: University of Chicago Press.

Hjelm, K., Bard, L., Berntorp, K., and Apelqvist, J. (2009). Beliefs about health and illness post-partum in women born in Sweden and the Middle East. *Midwifery*, *25*(5), 564–575.

Kaufman, S.R., and Fjord, L. (2011). Medicare, ethics, and reflexive longevity: governing time and treatment in an aging society. *Medical Anthropology Quarterly*, *25*(2), 209–231.

Kaufman, S.R., Russ, A.J., and Shim, J.K. (2006). Aged bodies and kinship matters: The ethical field of kidney transplant. *American Ethnologist*, *33*(1), 81–99.

Le Gall, J., and Cassan, C. (2010). Le point de vue des hommes immigrants sur leur non-utilisation des services de santé de première ligne. In A. Battaglini, ed., *Les services sociaux et de santé en contexte pluriethnique* (pp. 191–218). Montréal: Éditions Saint-Martin.

Le Gall, J., and Xenocostas, S. (2011). L'adaptation des soins à la diversité religieuse au Québec: L'exemple de la première ligne. *Ethnologie*, *33*(1), 169–189.

Le Gall, J., Montgomery, C., and Cassan, C. (2009). L'invisibilité de la participation des hommes immigrants dans les soins à leur famille. In M.E. Leandro, P.N. De Sousa Nossa, V.T. Rodrigues, and S. Sociedade, eds., *Os contributos (ub)visíveis da família* (pp. 73–95). Viseu: PsicoSoma.

Meintel, D., and Fortin, S. (2002). The new French fact. *Canadian Ethnic Studies*, *34*(3), 1–4.

Ny, P., Plantin, L., Dejin-Karlsson, E., and Dykes, A.-K. (2007). Middle Eastern mothers in Sweden, their experiences of the maternal health service and their partner's involvement. *Reproductive Health*, *4*, 1–9.

Ny, P., Plantin, L., Dejin-Karlsson, E., and Dykes, A.-K. (2008). The experience of Middle Eastern men living in Sweden of maternal and child health care and fatherhood: Focus-group discussions and content analysis. *Midwifery*, *24*, 281–290.

Pels, T. (2000). Muslim families from Morocco in the Netherlands: Gender dynamics and fathers' roles in a context of change. *Current Sociology*, *48*, 75–93.

Statistics Canada (2007). *Montreal (Québec): 2006 community profiles.* Retrieved from www. statcan.gc.ca.

Van der Geest, S., and Finkler, K. (2004). Hospital ethnography: Introduction. *Social Science & Medicine, 59*(10), 1995–2001.

Yount, K.M. (2006). Health and reproductive health: Overview. In S. Joseph, ed., *Encyclopedia of women & Islamic cultures: Vol. III, Family, body, sexuality and health* (pp. 211–218). Leiden, Netherlands: Brill.

Zaman, S. (2005). *Broken limbs, broken lives: Ethnography of a hospital ward in Bangladesh.* Amsterdam: Het Spinhuis.

8 'I am here not to repair but see the person as a whole'

Pastoral care work in German hospitals

Julia Thiesbonenkamp-Maag

Research methods

This contribution is based on research conducted on chaplains doing pastoral care in different hospitals all over Germany. The research team consists of two theologians (Fabian Kliesch, Thorsten Moos); one biologist, specializing in medical ethics (Simone Ehm); and one medical anthropologist (Julia Thiesbonenkamp-Maag). The study is part of an ongoing research project of the Protestant Institute for Interdisciplinary Research in Heidelberg that involves conducting expert interviews with hospital chaplains and carrying out participant observation in different hospitals. The names of the hospital chaplains as well as the hospital names used here are pseudonyms. As the community of hospital chaplains in Germany is tightly knit, this is one of way of ensuring anonymity for our interlocutors. The data presented here pertains to Protestant hospital chaplains if not stated otherwise. Before detailing the work of the hospital chaplains in this study, I will provide a brief overview of the historical background of pastoral care in Germany.

Pastoral care in Germany

Both the Protestant and the Catholic Church employ hospital chaplains in German hospitals. In general, they are carrying on a clerical tradition dating back to the Middle Ages, when poor people in the Western hemisphere sought (medical) care from monasteries. Medical care as well as moral and spiritual guidance were intertwined (Zaman, 2005, p. 6). Until the eighteenth century, hospitals 'were institutions of charity and welfare, and warehouses for the poor' (Van der Geest and Finkler, 2004, p. 1996). The modern hospital as we know it today was shaped by progress in the medical sciences, such as the development and provision of antiseptics (Van der Geest and Finkler, 2004, p. 1996). Part of this process was the continuing elaboration and differentiation of the medical sciences into different fields of speciality. During the twentieth century, knowledge about the psychological and psychosomatic contexts of diseases increased and new specialities evolved. One part of this evolution is the increasing professionalization of pastoral care over the last 35 years. The pastoral curriculum is based on theoretical and methodological concepts adopted from psychotherapy as well as clerical concepts from the guidelines of the Evangelical Church in Germany (EKD, 2004, p. 12).

Caring as an attitude

Although in the hospital today the focus is on medical objectives and the treatment of diseases and injuries (Norwood, 2006, p. 6), people in the hospital 'are more than their sicknesses', as one pastoral care worker stated. The pastoral care worker maintains relationships with patients, their relatives, and medical and administrative staff, but they often occupy a position at the fringe, so much so that one pastoral care worker used the metaphor of being 'an alien' as a description. The caring attitude adopted by chaplains is furthered by the fact that they try to hold themselves back (Norwood, 2006, pp. 19–20). One pastoral care worker said: 'I try to see the other. I try to see his or her hardship. Especially when I have a different point of view, I have to restrain myself. I have to be non-judgemental. Then we can have an open conversation.' This chaplain's words show that respect and mindfulness are two important aspects of care, values echoed again in the following statement:

> Some years ago I verbalized something like a guideline for my work. I think it is still true in a certain way. It is: 'Love is more important than truth'. This might sound very provocative. But I think, when you confront the patient with the truth, you can destroy him. If someone does not want to listen to certain things, you should not shout them at him. I see myself as a companion. I try to encourage and console them. I try to unburden them. A few weeks ago there was a woman who was supposed to get a new lung. But her condition dramatically deteriorated, so it was not possible to transplant the lung anymore. This patient said she wished she had made more journeys to foreign countries. She felt that she had missed out on something. But during our conversation she told me of one journey to Venice and Lake Garda. Her eyes lit up. It unburdened her and she recognized that she had not missed out on so much in her life. I think this made the process of dying easier for her. I understand myself as a birth attendant. To bring hidden things into the light.

The statements above illustrate that care is a complex concept interweaving different kinds of practices, emotions, and thoughts. Caring does not take place without power disparities. But, as seen in the statement above, care can empower, especially when the uniqueness of each person is recognized (Conradi, 2001, pp. 45–60). The theological approach to care, which focuses on the integration of the person, is similar to other psychological or philosophical traditions. Additionally, the theological approach includes spiritual or metaphysical dimensions of life (Yeates, 2009, p. 180; EKD, 2004). Generally, hospital chaplains try to strengthen the afflicted person, caring for the sick by listening and talking to them. Depending on the patient, they may also offer to pray and sing with them as a kind of spiritual care. The ministering of normal and special kinds of services is also part of their work. The aim is to enable patients to integrate their suffering into their lives (EKD, 2004, pp. 17–18).

Care as a practice

Norwood (2006, p. 3) states that chaplains' work 'includes a range of activities from the sacred to the profane'. The following vignettes serve to illustrate the point.

'Letter paper'

One day I was accompanying a chaplain named Ms. Christlieb during her daily rounds in the hospital. Ms. Christlieb works in a geriatric hospital, and about 80% of her time is spent caring for palliative patients. During our rounds, Ms. Christlieb told me that she had to remember to fetch some letter paper, explaining that it was for an old lady who was about to die. The patient wanted to write a letter to her little grandchildren so that they could read it when they were old enough, and remember their grandmother.

'Opening a sacred room'

'Opening a sacred room': these are the words of a Catholic pastoral care worker who had spent time with grieving parents in the hospital chapel, after they had lost their twins just after birth. She told me that it was very important to create a place where the parents could feel secure and peaceful—to not replicate the frantic behaviour of the medical staff, but to be calm and stable and 'project an engaged and available persona' (Norwood, 2006, p. 90). The chaplain offered the parents her time, giving them a chance to talk about their experiences with the twins. During that time the pastoral care worker had the feeling that time slowed down and the earth stood still. When they were unsure if the twins' older sibling should come to the hospital in order to say goodbye, she encouraged the parents to bring the sibling to the hospital. The chaplain stated that in times of crisis it is important that there is someone present who endures the pain with the people suffering, someone who offers to take the next few steps together with them.

Although these two examples are quite different—one act is rather profane while the other belongs to the sacred realm—they share some features. Both are ways of caring. Both hospital chaplains recognized needs. They did not reduce the patients to their symptoms but saw them as whole persons embedded in different kinds of social networks. Especially in the case of the deceased twins, the pastoral care worker bore witness, recognizing the twins as persons and acknowledging the metaphysical dimension.

Caring as witnessing

Pastoral care workers are not only witnesses for patients and their kin. They also bear witness to the work of doctors. For example, one day a chaplain named Ms. Fürst was asked to baptize and bless twins. One twin, Sophia, was severely impaired, while the other, Lisa, was smaller but healthy. Sophia's electroencephalogram (EEG) did not show any brain activity; she barely moved and was attached to a life support machine. The parents and the medical staff decided to remove Sophia from the life support machine and let her die. The day when Sophia was taken from the life support machine Ms. Fürst was there to bless her. Then something interesting happened, as this excerpt from an interview with her shows:

> The doctor entered the room. I was closer to the door than the parents. First the doctor turned towards me, but he did not look at me, which I found rather peculiar. Then he explained the medical condition of Sophia. He stated that the parents knew it and understood it. He also mentioned that the parents had agreed with his decision to take Sophia off the life support machine. I approved of this as I had asked the parents if it was OK for them to let their child die. Then the doctor said that the criterion of brain death does not work in the case of newborns. But the EEG that was run twice did show that the brain was severely damaged. He concluded that it was indicated to switch off the machine. Then he and a nurse took Sophia off the life support machine. The doctor waited until Sophia was dead.

Afterwards I understood that in my role as a hospital chaplain I was a kind of witness for the doctor. I think the doctor noticed that there was an ethical conflict. It was important for him to explain and justify his decision. It was also important for him that he could make sure that the parents understood what kind of decision they had taken.

This extract shows that care-as-witnessing is an attitude and a practice in which the hospital chaplain meets the person where she is (Norwood, 2006, pp. 19–20). It also exemplifies that hospital chaplains enter into relationships with patients and their kin, as well as medical staff.

Summary

Hospital chaplains relate to patients, their kin, and hospital staff in a manner that is informed by an ethos of care. Caring entails the dimension of practice as well as the emotional and spiritual level (Brückner and Thiersch, 2005, p. 138): chaplains recognize both the spiritual needs of people and the necessity of care as witnessing. Finally, their ethos of care is informed by understanding health in a holistic manner—as one said, 'not to repair, but to see the person as a whole'.

References

Brückner, M., and Thiersch, H. (2005). Care und Lebensweltorientierung. In W. Thole, P. Cloos, F. Ortmann, and V. Strutwolf, eds., *Soziale Arbeit im Öffentlichen Raum: Soziale Gerechtigkeit in der Gestaltung des Sozialen* (pp. 137–149). Wiesbaden: Verlag für Sozialwissenschaften.
Conradi, E. (2001). *Take Care: Foundations of an Ethics of Carefulness*. Frankfurt/M.: Campus.
EKD (2004). *Die Kraft zum Menschsein Stärken: Leitlinien für die Evangelische Kranken-hausseelsorge: Eine Orientierungshilfe*. Evangelische Kirche in Deutschland. Retrieved from https://www.ekd.de/download/leitlinien_krankenhausseelsorge_ekd_2004.pdf.
Norwood, F. (2006). The ambivalent chaplain: Negotiating structural and ideological difference on the margins of modern-day hospital medicine. *Medical Anthropology*, 25(2), 1–29.
Van der Geest, S., and Finkler, K. (2004). Hospital ethnography: Introduction. *Social Science & Medicine*, 59(10), 1995–2001.
Yeates, N. (2009). *Globalizing care economies and migrant workers: Explorations in global care chains*. New York: Palgrave Macmillan.
Zaman, S. (2005). *Broken limbs, broken lives: Ethnography of a hospital ward in Bangladesh*. Amsterdam: Het Spinhuis.

9   Palliative care at home in the case of ALS

Martine Verwey

The experience of family caregivers in end-of-life care and the potential for conflict in their relationships with healthcare professionals is largely uncharted territory. My current research in Switzerland focuses on the valuable perspective family caregivers can offer, particularly in home palliative care of amyotrophic lateral sclerosis (ALS) or motor neuron disease (MND) patients. Research into ALS is being conducted in many fields; the main area in which I am interested is the role of informal caregivers of patients living with ALS.

Since 2009 researchers in ALS genetics have identified several disease-causing genes.[1] Despite intensive research there are still no effective treatments to stop or reverse the course of this disease, which leads to death due to respiratory failure after an average of three to five years. People with ALS become severely disabled as the disease progresses. However, epidemiological studies show that both the rate of progression of the disease as well as survival rates vary considerably. ALS has an annual incidence rate of 2 per 100,000 and a prevalence of approximately 6–8 per 100,000. At any given time, approximately 700 people are living with ALS in Switzerland, 1000 in the Netherlands, 5000 in the UK, 6000 in Germany, and as many as 30,000 in the United States. It is not its prevalence that legitimizes this chronic disorder as the focus of research, but rather the high level of practical,

---

1   This ever-increasing pace of new discoveries is giving people with ALS hope for a cure; at the same time it raises expectations and urges health-seeking activities. Ene (2009) highlights how shared ALS identity empowers members of the community to take action against the disease. However, both scientists and the people affected are well aware that translating laboratory research to therapies for humans takes time, and facing this insight if you are living with ALS yourself requires inner strength. In the case of ALS, the increasing gap between diagnostics and therapeutics noted by Rabinow (1996) is painfully true. Despite promising genetic discoveries, this chronic progressive neuromuscular disorder is terminal. A complex interplay between genetic susceptibility and environmental exposure is, according Chad et al. (2013), likely to be important in the pathogenesis of ALS. Coordinating with patient groups in the early stages of clinical studies and encouraging dialogue between patients and study investigators is a strongly advocated approach to help identify specific causes of the disease (Chad et al., 2013). The ALS community, as shown by Mitsumoto and Turner (2013), is actively engaged in carrying out therapeutic trials.

cognitive, emotional, and spiritual challenges placed upon ALS patients and their families.

Research objectives

While ALS is a terminal illness, I am more intrigued by the ways of thinking about the terminally ill than by the euthanasia discourse related to the disease. Interventions upon life and understandings of life include interventions upon death and understandings of death. At which moment does life lose its potential value? This interest is grounded in my personal experiences caring for my late husband. As the author, my position is twofold: as the former primary caregiver for my lifelong partner and as an anthropologist. My goal is to contribute to the optimization of care by studying how family members can best be supported in providing care at home. At the same time I aim to bring clarification to ways of acting upon dying. The main research questions are: What constitutes 'good care' at home for patients with ALS? How can or should family caregivers and health professionals work together to make it happen?

Medical gaze and reification

In this section, to go deeper into ways of dealing with terminal illness, I refer to 'memory minutes', observations, and a selection of sketches of health professionals in action published in Verwey (2010). To be ill with ALS means that one can no longer rely on the security of the familiar functions provided by the body over the years; one must find a way to adapt to disablement. Neurologists assure their patients that there is much evidence of 'stable phases' occurring during the course of the illness, times when the progression of the illness seems to halt. However, the process of adaptation can be so demanding that a person living with ALS needs a great deal of strength not to abandon hope that such stabilization is possible. As a member of a close family, I rather longed for this, but hardly dared to believe it possible.

> While my partner was still able to travel, against the advice of some disbelieving professional caregivers in our town in Switzerland, we often made long journeys by train through France and the Netherlands. It meant freedom and it gave us strength, knowing that in spite of everything we were still capable of intense enjoyment. After a lengthy summer absence,

we were visited by the physiotherapist who had treated my husband in her practice at the beginning and later, with the advancing illness, at home. 'Have there been any new developments?' she asked, as usual. Her client stood smiling in front of her and answered: 'Stabilization.' It was his way of referring to the welcomed plateau that had lasted three months that summer. The physiotherapist had not seen him for a while and was no longer used to his speech, which had been deteriorating. 'What?' she asked. Meanwhile, I had placed myself alongside the therapist and could observe the situation. The client repeated quietly, with a broad smile: 'Stabilization.' The therapist still did not understand him, and asked, 'What do you mean?' For the third time the client, still smiling broadly, replied: 'Stabilization.' Abruptly, the therapist turned her head to me and said, 'Speech doesn't function anymore either.'

This encounter exemplifies the process of reification or the transformation from subject into object. The importance of maintaining a personal, human relationship is stressed over and over in disability studies, as I have shown (Verwey, 2010). The production of a 'medical gaze' (Foucault, 1973) can be avoided, as has been documented by Pols (2005) in her research of long-term mental healthcare in the Netherlands, in which she analyses communication practices between nurses and patients. She highlights a concrete situation where a patient is treated as a subject by the nurses, and she concludes that the patient in this situation 'is not objectified as being determined by a medical condition, however ill he may be' (Pols, 2005, p. 212). A focus on a patient as 'the other'—or as an object—in which they are perceived as dominated by a medical condition harms a disabled person (Verwey, 2010).

Change in attitude towards a terminally ill person

As my partner became weaker and increasingly reliant on the help of others, I noticed now and then a different approach by professionals, one that was more technical and less personal. It has been established that informal caregivers, most often spouses or close family members, play a central role in the patient's well-being (Wasner, 2008). Humour and attention are needed as much as technical care. Therefore, it appears to be extremely important for caregivers to be given sufficient information on the illness, its course, terminal conditions, practical help options, and technical interventions. Understandably, palliative care specialists are keen to prevent burnout in family caregivers.

As long as it was still possible, I took advantage of opportunities to take a few days off and rest. In my absence, friends, neighbours, and professionals took over the necessary care during the day and through the night. As the illness progressed and care became more complex, the palliative care physician and palliative homecare nurse increasingly spoke of a possible short stay in a hospice for my partner, even if only for one day. My husband and I knew that the stress of the transfer would outweigh the benefits of the rest for me as primary caregiver. These discussions with palliative care specialists frequently had undercurrents of tension. Once the general practitioner made it clear to me that I must take an afternoon off on a regular basis and should enlist the help of home healthcare assistants. In answer to my objection that too often my husband's needs and requirements were overlooked and that we therefore preferred professional caregivers, the GP commented to my husband: 'Well, then just sit uncomfortably for a few hours.' On another occasion, during an endless assessment and a strained discussion about staying in a hospice once a week, the palliative homecare nurse said irritably, 'In that case, Mr. S. will just have to bite the bullet [using the German phrase 'bite a sour apple'].'[2]

In the communication between my husband and myself from then on, we had only to spell out the words 'sour apple' and I knew that I had tried to do something against his will. In certain situations, if he indicated the letter 'S', we both just broke into laughter. Thus the nurse's comment became our slogan of resistance. No doubt indeed, burnout prevention in family caregivers is most important, but below the surface a serious change in attitude towards a terminally ill person might be brewing.[3]

Considering suicide as a way of dealing with terminal illness

At which moment does life lose its potential value? At which point does the biovalue of a terminally ill person start deteriorating? Shortly after my husband passed away, his respiratory physician said to me, 'I don't

2   'Herr S. muss dann halt in den sauren Apfel beissen'.
3   Lock (2008, p. 63) elaborates referring to Novas and Rose (2000) on an emerging 'mutation in personhood' based on the results of recent advances in the life sciences, including human genetics and genetic medicine, and partly instigated by social categories and classifications. Stigma has a lot to do with social classifications. Can a change in approach towards a terminally ill person losing strength be explained by a mutation in the perception of this person?

understand why more people with ALS don't commit suicide in Switzerland. Instead, they take a chance, and then we have a situation where someone ends up being overburdened, as in your case.' Had my partner and I evaded the subject of ending life voluntarily? Days after the definite diagnosis, our general practitioner asked my husband whether he would consider suicide as a possible way of dealing with his terminal illness. He would not, he said, 'out of respect towards life', as he told me afterwards. In his Advance Decision to Refuse Treatment (preferences for medical decisions at the end of life) his wish for no life-sustaining treatment had been documented. But didn't we think beyond the written advance care directives? Were we reluctant to deal with the subject? Did we suppress the inevitable?

Half a year before my lifelong partner died, I spoke on the telephone with the palliative care physician regarding medication; it was a few days before Easter. During the talk he suddenly asked me whether my husband had ever said he'd had enough of life. Astonished, and without the slightest doubt, I answered: 'No.' The physician then explained that in the event my partner ever expressed the wish to die, this could be considered. I asked the physician whether in that case he would assist him. He said he was not permitted to, but there were viable alternatives aside from organizations for assisted suicide. At that time, my husband was neither able to raise his arms nor swallow, and I realized that I was the one who would actively have to assist him in euthanasia and would afterwards have to live with the knowledge of my action. The physician ended the conversation by requesting that I discuss the subject with my partner during the Easter holidays. Several days went by before I found the courage to tell my husband about the phone call with the physician, and to ask him directly whether he wished to end his life. Quietly and clearly he indicated that he did not. Easter passed calmly, without worries. We suspected it would be our last together.

More than two years had passed between this phone call with the palliative care physician and the moment of definite diagnosis, when the general practitioner first raised the question of considering suicide. In the course of advancing illness, the inner state of mind can change radically with regard to suicide, and it is therefore important that the physician try to ascertain what the patient is considering and what his needs and requirements are. Raising the question of suicide on the phone could lead to misunderstanding, as the suggestion may be received by the terminally ill patient as a reduction of his or her life to an economic and emotional burden.

Reflection

The aforementioned tensions can be very well explained by a divergence of perspectives noted by Brown (2003) between healthcare professionals and people living with ALS. As Sakellariou et al. (2013) have illustrated in their review on experiences of people living with ALS, medical care tries to balance between what is good for one world and what for another. Patients, their next of kin, and health professionals live in worlds separated from one another. In palliative care at home, they depend on one another and on communicating to each other their goals and needs. Only a combination of quality standards for 'good care' and expertise as well as respect for patients' self-determination will do justice to the complex situation of ALS palliative care at home.

References

Brown, J.B. (2003). User, carer and professional experiences of care in motor neurone disease. *Primary Health Care and Development*, 4(3), 207–217.

Chad, D.A., et al. (2013). Funding agencies and disease organizations: Resources and recommendations to facilitate ALS clinical research. *Amyotrophic Lateral Sclerosis and Frontotemporal Degeneration*, 14(Suppl. 1), 62–66.

Ene, S. (2009). Biosocial communities: Community participation in public health. In *Public health management & policy: An on-line textbook*, 12th ed. Retrieved from the Case Western Reserve University website: http://www.cwru.edu/med/epidbio/mphp439/Biosocial_Comm.pdf.

Foucault, M. (1973). *The birth of the clinic: An archaeology of medical perception*. London: Tavistock.

Mitsumoto, H., and Turner, M.R. (2013). Promoting clinical and patient-oriented research to identify the pathogenesis of amyotrophic lateral sclerosis. *Amyotrophic Lateral Sclerosis and Frontotemporal Degeneration*, 14(Suppl. 1), 1–4.

Lock, M. (2008). Biosociality and susceptibility genes: A cautionary tale. In S. Gibbon and C. Novas, eds., *Biosocialities, genetics and the social sciences: Making biologies and identities* (pp. 56–78). New York: Routledge.

Novas, C., and Rose, N. (2000). Genetic risk and the birth of the somatic individual. *Economy and Society*, 29, 485–513.

Pols, J. (2005). Enacting appreciations: Beyond the patient perspective. *Health Care Analysis*, 13(3), 203–221.

Rabinow, P. (1996). Artificiality and enlightenment: From sociobiology to biosociality. In P. Rabinow, ed., *Essays on the anthropology of reason* (pp. 91–111). Princeton: Princeton University Press.

Sakellariou, D., Boniface, G., and Brown, P. (2013). Experiences of living with motor neurone disease: A review of qualitative research. *Disability and Rehabilitation*, 35(21), 1765–1773.

Verwey, M. (2010). Proximity and distance in palliative care from the perspective of primary caregiver. *Medische Antropologie*, 22(1), 31–46.

Wasner, M. (2008). Resilienz bei Patienten mit amyotropher Lateralsklerose (ALS) und ihren Angehörigen. *Schweizer Archiv für Neurologie und Psychiatrie*, 159(8), 500–505.

10   Configurations for action

How French general practitioners handle their patients'
consumption of psychotropic drugs

Claudie Haxaire

Ehrenberg declares in *La fatigue d'être soi* (The fatigue of being oneself,
1998, p. 249) that depression and addiction are two figures of contemporary
subjectivity, with addiction being a way to fight depression, according to
psychiatrists. The author puts forward the hypothesis that depression is
'a pathology of a society where the norm is no longer based on guilt and
discipline, but on initiative. [...] [T]he individual is therefore faced with a
pathology of inadequacy. [...] [T]he depressed person is a person who has
broken down', and 'addiction is nostalgia for a lost subject'.

Addiction to commonly consumed substances such as alcohol and
tobacco, or to illegal products (cannabis, heroin, cocaine), also occurs with
psychotropic drugs. In France—the country with the highest consumption
of psychotropic drugs in Europe (Briot, 2006)—antidepressants, hypnotic
drugs, and minor tranquilizers figure on the list of pharmaceuticals requiring a doctor's prescription. In 80% of cases the prescriber is the general
practitioner (GP) who also plays a preventive role in public health, diagnos-
ing and treating the abuse of legal nonpharmaceutical psychotropics and
illicit substances by prescribing substitute products, if necessary. These
cases are part of the complexity of the GP's practice, and notably the social
aspect of primary care, described as a 'bio-psycho-social' practice by the
World Organization of Family Doctors (WONCA) (Allen et al., 2002). The GPs
who work with these new subjectivities are hence also and simultaneously
actors in their construction.

In our studies of consumers' understanding of psychotropic drugs (Haxaire
et al., 2005) we have shown that these drugs fall into the category of medication that 'calms the nerves' like other psychotropics; they are managed within
the personal private sphere. For consumers, and counter to all expectations,
these drugs are not part of the world of medicine. In these circumstances,
how can their doctors—practitioners dealing with these pathologies that
'list the different facets of intimate unhappiness' (Ehrenberg, 1998)—handle
the use of psychotropic drugs in the broadest sense?

The study presented here is a new analysis of data previously gathered
in the collective project I conducted, 'Addictive Behaviour Management of

Outpatients by Western Brittany GPs', which was published in Haxaire et al. (2003). This new analysis shows that where psychotropics are concerned GPs modulate their care depending on the most urgent need—sometimes social, sometimes medical—in short, according to the context, or, as I will show, the 'configuration' of the problem as perceived by the GP at a particular point in their relationship with the patient. It also demonstrates that GPs are implicated in different ways in these configurations, and that the psychotropic substances have varying significance, depending on whether taking the drugs into account means crossing a line of privacy, a historically variable boundary that is also characteristic of the contemporary society that shapes our subjectivity (Elias, 1973). I use the term 'configuration' here in its ordinary meaning (the set of characteristics of a system or overall characteristics), and not as the concept proposed by Elias (1970) to signify that society is a network of interdependency between individuals. However, it is indeed the relational reasoning recommended by Elias and taken up by Ehrenberg (2010) that casts light on the practices discussed in this study.

Methodology

To grasp the practical knowledge of GPs the project constructed a survey inspired by principles of ethnomethodology (Garfinkel, 1967). This survey was used to collect GPs' 'accounts'[1] of their encounters in a given day, as narrated in their offices to the author.[2] The doctors reported on their practices for a day chosen randomly, in a week during which they filled out a table tracking their practice. The respondents were asked to report any issues of dependency related to their consultations. The 'accounts' were recorded and later transcribed.

One particular modification of the survey protocol should be noted here. While the table tracking each GP's practice covered an entire week, only the consultations of the randomly chosen day were to be discussed in detail (restricted corpus: D=day). But as the first doctor interviewed wanted to comment on substitutive treatments for patients seen on other days, the protocol was modified to include comments on consultations held throughout the week (unrestricted corpus: W=week). This unrestricted

---

1   According to Garfinkel (1967), the main property of practical knowledge is 'accountability'.
2   The author is an anthropologist who was initially trained as a pharmacist, and therefore shares doctors' assumptions to some extent.

corpus proved valuable because it enables us to see the full range of concerns (the 'operational category') in which the GPs include issues related
to psychotropics.

With a panel of ten GPs in western France (five in rural areas and
five practicing in a small town)[3] we compiled 968 consultations (46 days
of office visits). GPs reported in detail on 209 consultations from the
randomly chosen day; additional comments were offered on 144 consultations among the remaining 759 consultations. The entire corpus of
data on which the analysis is based is thus made up of comments on 353
consultations.

For our analysis we initially applied a substance-by-substance approach
that turned out to be limited, as it did not allow us to grasp the GPs' practices. We then applied a semiological analysis using ALCESTE, a textual
data analysis software program,[4] which showed the different attitudes of
the GPs regarding their patients' habits. These attitudes were not linked to
the particular type of substance, but a clear distinction appears between
the encounters in which the GP focused on medical problems and merely
listed psychotropic medication, and those in which the psychotropics were
handled in different ways depending on the mode and circumstances of
consumption reported by the patient.

This semiological analysis led me to re-examine the data and reclas-
sify the GP consultation reports by type of response to the patient's
consumption of psychotropics (whether known to the GP or not), and
by the reasoning behind these responses, depending on the patient's
circumstances and the therapeutic relationship at the time. I call these
reactions 'configurations for action', which are presented in the typology
below.

3   The sample of GPs was diverse, in terms of practice, outpatients, and age, but corresponds
to an average profile according to health insurance data for the Brittany region (Haxaire et al.,
2003).
4   The ALCESTE software, designed by M. Reinert, is applied to a body of text to extract classes
of enunciations that are related by their vocabulary, called 'lexical worlds'. Reinert (1992, 1993)
hypothesizes that 'at the time of locution the speaker invests various successive worlds, and
these worlds, in imposing their objects at the same time impose their vocabulary. Consequently,
a statistical study of the distribution of this vocabulary should enable us to pick up the trace of
these "mental spaces" that the speaker has successively inhabited, traces that are perceptible in
terms of "lexical worlds", these lexical worlds referring back to a way of choosing one reference
system or another, at a given moment in the discourse'.

General practitioners and psychotropics: Configurations for action, and the place and handling of products in these configurations

When reviewing the consumption of psychotropics by their patients, the doctors could not isolate each type of product, nor distinguish the relationship to these products from the context in which they were consumed (for example, partying or trying to relieve tension). The products themselves are less important than how they are taken and in what context. Consumption of certain products (tobacco, cannabis, and also alcohol) is not taken into account if they do not raise concerns or create tension, in relation to the problems that the doctor is treating.

In most consultations, GPs neither intervene in patients' consumption of psychotropics, nor mention them as such, because they feel they have nothing to say about it (i.e., no problem is clearly apparent), or, on the contrary, in configurations 7 and 8 (see table below), because they are overwhelmed by the medical or psychiatric gravity of the presenting problem (whether it is related to the consumption of psychotropic substances or not). In a discourse analysis, personal pronouns corresponding the patient/GP relationship are not included; what is mentioned is the state of the patient and their condition from the GP's description (Haxaire et al., 2003).

When GPs do mention them as such and intervene (or not, as in configuration 3), they are focused on their patient, and positioned to interact with patients (configurations 3, 4, 5, and 6). Discourse is taken over by the GP: they refer to the GP/patient dyad as 'we' and they restate moments of communication with them. GPs may be worried about consumption that they perceive as self-medication for the problems they are trying to treat, but they do not attempt to replace these substances because, in their diagnosis, the patient needs them (configuration 3). GPs might also focus on their patient's personal problems, by listening to them or prescribing psychotropic drugs (configuration 4), or by trying to reduce their social isolation (due to addictive behaviour or psychotic problems) with prescriptions of buprenorphine or tiapride (configuration 5). They might also attempt to contain the crises that overwhelm the patient (configuration 6). But sometimes it emerges that the patient does not consume psychotropics, revealing a configuration that is a negative imprint, where the GP feels the patient *should* be taking psychotropics (configuration 9).

Table 1 Summary of the 'configurations' and the percentage of the consultation accounts in each category

No GP action on psychotropic consumption (posture: focus on medical issue)					GP action on psychotropic consumption (posture: interaction with patient)				Waiting for action
Nothing to say 49.5%			Overwhelmed by gravity 21%		Prescribed medication	Prescribed medication	Prescribed substitute	Prescribed medication	Negative imprint
0 – 'No prob-lem'	1 – 'No depen-dency'	2 – 'No depen-dency but…'	7 – Medical gravity	8 – Psy-chiatric gravity	3 – Self-medica-tion 'He needs it'	4 – Non-normal use but self-medication	5 – Focus on social issue	6 – Crisis that over-whelmed the patient	9 – 'Patient should have it'
33%	14%	2.5%	10%	11%	14.5%	3.5%	4%	6%	1.5%

Nothing to be envisioned in the way of action

In slightly over half of the consultations for which comments were mandatory no action is planned in relation to any psychotropic substance.

Configuration 0—'No problem'.[5] In most of these cases the possibility of action did not even occur to the doctor. But their comments ('no particular problem' or 'apparently no problem') shed light on the specific feature of this configuration. In order for a doctor to look for any kind of dependency, he or she must perceive a problem, or must be informed of it, even though it cannot be assumed that a problem is absent: 'As far as I know, there is no problem.' In this configuration these behaviours, if they exist, are entirely confined to the private sphere. They are neither communicated to nor perceived by the practitioner. They are considered to be beyond the doctor's scope, even though the practitioner knows of the possibility of them, and the practitioner has decided to focus on his/her own field, biomedical issues.

Configuration 1—'No dependency, or in any case it wasn't mentioned', 'doesn't smoke, doesn't drink'. In fewer cases the issue is considered via a negation. GPs either mention dependency in general or enumerate behaviours ('doesn't smoke, doesn't drink', or, less frequently, 'doesn't take drugs'), to which they may or may not add consumption of psychotropic drugs ('no sleeping pills, no drugs') prescribed by the doctors themselves.[6] Nothing here pushes the doctor to look for a dependency problem, and the doctor can't be sure, or hasn't asked directly, because nothing hints at dependency.

In the eyes of the doctors alcohol and tobacco are the prototypical substances that can induce dependency. While the consumption of certain substances can be deduced by the doctor because they interact negatively with the patient's pathology, it is not always easy to be sure that there is no dependency or moderate consumption of common psychotropics, such as alcohol. The doctors cannot be certain, as reflected in comments such

5   The 504 consultations in the weekly corpus that were not commented on would likely fall into this category, but we must take into consideration that some doctors were in a greater hurry than others, and so we cannot be sure.

6   It is no longer a matter of 'particular problems', as these are manifested in the addictive behaviours, but of these behaviours alone seen in a medical perspective, without mentioning a context that justifies them, because the behaviours weren't brought to light. The word 'dependency' seems to reflect a medical attitude. An analysis by substance shows that this is not the case, however, as the practitioners do not use the diagnostic tools available to them in the case of alcohol consumption, for example.

as, 'in any case I have never observed it'. In order to break down possible
dependency behaviours substance by substance, or to diagnose a particular
behaviour, this behaviour must differ markedly from ordinary behaviour,
must show a 'sign', must stand out from the private sphere. In some cases,
GPs relate the non-consumption of psychotropics to 'psychological' traits:
'Nothing, nothing else on the psychological level. She doesn't drink, doesn't
smoke, and—that's all.'

The fact that consumption of psychotropic drugs, medically prescribed,
appears in this comment: 'It's the same, there's no dependency, whether
tobacco, alcohol, sleeping pills, or medicines', shows that GPs are aware of
the regulating role they are supposed to play. But as far as drugs 'for sleep'
are concerned, it should be noted that the practitioners often seemed to
have forgotten what they have prescribed, and have to check their patients'
files. It is as if, in the specific tension of this configuration, the medical act
of prescribing a drug 'for sleep' is sucked into the private sphere.[7] Drugs 'for
sleep' are thus integrated into the domain of private life, the intimate in
the meaning ascribed by Elias; this is even more forcefully demonstrated
in the following configuration.

Configuration 2—'Doesn't smoke, doesn't drink, doesn't take medicine,
except...'. In nine instances, and exclusively in the D corpus, this enumera-
tion of potentially addictive behaviours, which is meant to show that they
are absent, ends up by either noting the presence of such behaviour, which
is minimized by contrast, or by characterizing the consumption of an addictive substance without a state of dependency.[8] In this configuration, a
patient's request for a hypnotic is minimized: 'doesn't drink, doesn't smoke,
doesn't take medicine, except for a little hypnotic'. The doctors surveyed
appear to feel that they have to justify these prescriptions, either by the
gravity of the pathology or the treatment of symptoms, or by mentioning
'passing' worries or events in the patient's life that lead to an equally 'passing' consumption of the psychotropic substance, without dependency.

Here we have a focus on the ordinary in the medical consultation; the
psychotropic substance (anxiolytic, hypnotic) is not a problem; on the
contrary, it is justified by the life context that is then referenced. The essential point is that there is no dependency: the patient doesn't smoke or

---

7   This is attested by the expressions used by the doctors, which were the same as those used
by the patients, with very few exceptions.
8   Food excesses are also added to this list, associated or not with the consumption of common
psychotropics.

drink excessively, or unspoken consumption is masked: 'he undoubtedly was once a heavy drinker'. The negative formulation 'not a psych problem' appears several times (also in the W corpus), suggesting that dependency on psychotropics is included in the category of 'psych problems', a point discussed below.

Recognition of dependency or unusual consumption: The GP is an actor, managing or channelling behaviour by prescribing psychotropic pharmaceuticals (focused on patient or social context)

When practitioners talk about the consumption of psychotropics that they treat, they speak not about the nature of the substance, but rather the context or the 'reasons' that the GPs attribute to this consumption, and they are clearly focused on the patient.

Configuration 3—Consumption as self-medication, complemented with medical treatment. The consumption of psychotropics, whether alcohol, tobacco, or hashish, poses a problem only when it reveals an underlying problem that the GPs seek to treat. They perceive the consumption of psychotropics as self-medication. The doctors focus on the patient and her/his social and 'psychological' context, insofar as treatment in the vein of 'psychological therapy' can help reduce the impact of the consumption of psychotropics, tobacco, hashish, and even narcotics; they also justify prescribing anxiolytics for someone 'who smokes some dope, but doesn't drink'.

This reasoning holds for narcotics when the doctor does not consider the subject to be an addict. One doctor said about a patient:

> He probably has done some heroin, maybe a little cocaine, but he's not a drug addict, he drinks a lot, huh. [...] This is a guy with pretty phenomenal physical strength who needs to expend his energy, and he came to see me this week, Friday. He told me he wanted to take Xanax again because he was all worked up in the morning, when life was too calm, when there wasn't much happening at work, he had a sort of energy. [...] He's been in some pretty rough situations, he likes that. So we got to talking about that [...] but he told me 'but I'm not going to drink a glass a whisky, OK—I need something to calm me down, otherwise I'm going to slug my boss', he tells me [laughing]; it's to relieve the pressure.

Sometimes this patient's doctor is willing to stabilize him by prescribing a 'little' psychotropic medication.

But most often the diagnosis is a depression disorder—'the depressive nature that I associate with alcohol consumption'; 'from one day to the next, out of the blue, she stopped smoking [and came to see me, depressed]'— and gives rise to treatment with an antidepressant. And thus alcohol and tobacco consumption are linked to depression and treated as such, with antidepressants. Benzodiazepine, when associated with an antidepressant treatment, can itself act as a substitute, despite the antidepressant, when the patient cannot deal with a personal experience, the death of a friend or family member, for example.

But the situation can call for more serious intervention—'We are well aware of what can come of it when it is associated with disorders, psychiatric disorders and heavy use of cannabis, like that'—leading to the young man who 'has blown a fuse' being referred to a 'psych colleague'. Cannabis is taken into account, considered a problem, only when it is accompanied by behavioural disorders, and then in the context of the interaction between the patient, his mother, and another doctor, psychologist, or psychiatrist.

It is not the substance itself that is important, but what is revealed by its consumption. This falls within the doctor's purview, and he/she treats it with an antidepressant or refers the patient to mental health services. In this configuration the doctors complement or replace the patients' psychotropic self-medication with a medical treatment, generally with medications that they deem to be more appropriate and less harmful.

Configuration 4—Non-normal consumption of possibly addictive psychoactive medications, to handle psychological problems. Dosages of pharmaceutical psychotropics need to be adjusted for elderly patients and in the presence of multiple pathologies, or when there is a risk of suicide, for example.

> So. For me, yes, it's her treatment. I asked her, she was in such a state of anxiety I asked her to stop taking the Xanax and she took Tranxene 50, a half a pill three times a day, a dose she could double if needed... So, there is really a major pathology. This woman can come in, in the midst of an anxiety attack, and sooner or later will commit suicide. I wouldn't say that she's not going to do it.

Managing psychotropic medications is the lot of GPs, whether they are juggling psychiatric treatments, antipain medication, or treatment of symptoms. They held concerns related to psychotropics, specifically, managing the balance between the risks of decompensation and dependency, whether in treatment or in the use of non-medical psychotropics. Within this configuration, GPs do not see dependency on medications as a problem; the important thing is to give care to the patient. The doctors are actors (they speak in the first person) and close to their patients, but still adopt a bit of distance by chuckling when recounting the 'reasons' for the suffering that is treated. The GPs are well aware that only medical care authorizes them to violate the patients' privacy in giving those reasons.

Configuration 5—Integration/non-integration: social issues are the priority. Heroin substitution treatment using Subutex (buprenorphine) is not considered problematic when it contributes to the social stabilization sought by the prescribing doctors. Because the GPs want to see their patients reintegrated into society they take the trouble to pursue difficult relationships with patients under opiate substitution therapy, and accordingly they report on the ups and downs of this reintegration, emphasizing the social problems and their solutions. They often wanted to talk about the ways in which they handled social issues in the cases where they were striving for social integration; the GPs commented on fifteen cases in the W corpus and only three in the D corpus, drawing upon all the patients of the week in order to discuss this topic, and their successes. The same is true for dependency on codeine-based analgesics that may allow people to maintain some sort of social life, and for elderly patients treated with neuroleptics.

Configuration 6—Compulsive behaviour of patient who is unable to cope. GPs also wanted to talk about patients who suffer from bouts of compulsive consumption. If the patient is in a crisis and cannot control his/her behaviour, the doctors take an active role and attempt to re-establish a balance for the patient. In this configuration they are aware of the problem and see it as part of their responsibility to address. Patients may manifest compulsive consumption of alcohol, tobacco, medications, surgery, or more, but once again it is not the substance itself that is important, but the behaviour. In this configuration, however, the doctors feel that the behaviour can be modified, because they continue to have an adequate relationship with their patients. Naturally they feel personally targeted by the crisis behaviour that gets out of hand ('he did this or that TO ME') but the diagnosis is enunciated in medical terms ('a recurring problem with alcohol'), showing the doctor's respect for *his/her* patient. When other doctors are mentioned the GPs are always acting for the patient's benefit. Knowing their patients, the doctors maintain the relationship ('she revealed that to ME, she told ME'), and they situate the compulsion in the life context as they know it, and think they can have an effect—they continue to be actors. When doctors address substance consumption, it is generally because they envision suitable medical or substitutive treatment, as if medication alone allowed them to intrude on their patients' privacy.

The doctor takes no action because the situation is beyond the scope of action

In this set of configurations, substances are mentioned but GPs do not act or do not think that they can act because the obvious psychiatric pathologies or serious somatic pathologies (eventually linked to consumption of alcohol or tobacco) are more than they can handle. The substances may be mentioned in colloquial and even slang terms ('she's a lush') but consumption is not often quantified.

Configuration 7—A psychiatric problem is more than the GP can handle. In the D corpus there are five instances of doctors reporting that they were confronted with psychiatric problems that were too much for them to handle. Sometimes current psychotropics are not mentioned, as if the psychiatric treatments alone were a reason to comment on the consultation, reinforcing the notion that consumption of psychotropics is linked to psychological/psychiatric issues. Here the doctors focus on the psychiatric problem.

Interaction with the patient is not noted; one of the GPs distances himself ('I am implicated without getting too involved'.).[9] If alcohol is mentioned, it is in the context of the psychiatric problem, or, in a subsidiary fashion, because the family is marked by alcohol consumption. The addictions are described using commonplace and even slang vocabulary.

Configuration 8—A serious pathology is more than the GP can handle. The doctors report an equal number of times in each corpus that they do not intervene in the consumption of psychotropics because the medical problems exceed the consumption problems, for example, in the case of cirrhosis. There may or may not be negotiations regarding the toxic substance, but the core issue is the serious somatic lesion: it is a matter of the patient's survival. Dependency is evoked with cautious wording ('I think', 'I believe').

---

9   The doctors tend to refer to classes of psychotropic drugs, or to list drugs by brand name, without specifications, which are signs of distance and non-appropriation of the psychiatrists' prescriptions that are frequently renewed.

The doctors are not in an interactive relationship with the patient. The gravity of related pathologies, or [the gravity] of the pathologies induced by substance consumption, generally alcohol, place the issue beyond the scope of dependent behaviour.[10] The doctors' accounts are neutral, bare-bones reports of their actions.

Upstream from the substances

Configuration 9—Configuration without substance: No particular dependency, no addiction, or psychotropic drugs to avoid, 'but the patient is suffering'. Three times in the unrestricted corpus (W) (and twice in the D corpus), consultations appear in which there is no mention of consumption of psychotropics, either commonplace substances or medications. The GPs relate the 'reasons' they believe that the patient is suffering, and will undoubtedly require prescription of psychotropic drugs or self-medication in the future, as exemplified in this statement: 'In any case she is definitely suffering. I don't know at all, but I have never prescribed anything—anyway, she is certainly a candidate to have something someday.' In this configuration the psychotropic appears only in its absence, and the patient is flagged as a 'psych' patient.

Here we find patients who present somatic-like conditions that are qualified as psychological: 'They don't use psychotropics, but they could, they should'. This negative configuration is important, because it effectively reveals the GPs' preoccupation with relating somatic and psychological conditions. If these consultations are found in the corpus it is precisely because psychic suffering is the problem outlined by the context. The GPs do not appear to be sure of what they are saying: they use an indefinite 'patient who', and upon occasion their laughter indicates a distance in relation to the gravity of the issue that worries them.

Conclusion

Analysis of these 'configurations of action', describing the steps taken by GPs with respect to consumption of various substances, underscores the weight of the doctor's knowledge of the patient's social context in the therapeutic

---

10   In some cases the patients are treated with antidepressants, without the doctor giving reasons for this prescription or relating the events in the patient's life that led them to make this decision.

decision. In most cases the 'reasons' given for prescribing, not prescribing, not intervening at all, or considering prescribing refer to

maintaining or restoring social integration (illustrated in an exemplary but non-specific way by prescription of buprenorphine or Subutex). These are indeed contextual 'reasons', if we refer to Wittgenstein's (1982) distinction between causes and reasons. This underscores the comprehensive posture that is induced by the biological, psychological, and social approach that is typical of GPs' medical care.

In these consultations consumption of psychoactive substances may be highlighted, seen as significant and requiring attention, or ignored. The nature of the psychotropic substance is more or less irrelevant. A significant proportion of this consumption falls outside of the doctors' field of vision because it is in the sphere of private life. When GPs consider intervening, it is often only to substitute a psychotropic medication for the original substance. Thus they adopt a medical position that is the only posture allowing them to intrude on their patients' private lives. Elias (1973) drew attention to the historically variable boundaries of intimacy, seen here again in an updated example of practices related to psychotropic drugs as tools for shaping contemporary subjectivity.

But this is not Elias's only contribution to our discussion.

These reports by GPs contain medical information—information on the patients, their state of well-being or unhappiness, their family background, and their social circumstances—documenting multiple points of tension. Each report gives precedence to one or another of these points, reflecting what has been targeted by the GP's intervention at this specific moment in time, even if the doctor, as family physician, has a global view of the situation. The relational approach proposed by Ehrenberg can be used to describe the interdependence of the different registers of tension; these form configurations that simultaneously determine and reflect the specific interaction of doctor and patient in the consultation. But these interactions are themselves contained in, and are reflections of, our contemporary society, normalized by specific societal modes that in turn are reinforced by the interactions. These specific interactions thus constitute the social configuration, as construed by Elias (1970), from which emerge the figures of contemporary subjectivity that are depression and addiction.

References

Allen, J., et al. (2002). The European definitions of the key features of the discipline of general practice: The role of the GP and core competencies. *British Journal of General Practice*, *52*(479), 526–527.

Briot, M. (2006). *Rapport sur le bon usage des médicaments psychotropes*. French National Assembly Report No. 3187. Retrieved from http://www.assemblee-nationale.fr/12/pdf/rap-off/i3187.pdf.

Ehrenberg, A. (1998). *La fatigue d'être soi: Dépression et société*. Paris: Odile Jacob.

Ehrenberg, A. (2010). *La société du malaise*. Paris: Odile Jacob.

Elias, N. (1970). *Qu'est-ce que la sociologie?* Paris: Poche Pocket.

Elias, N. (1973). *La civilisation des mœurs*. Paris: Calman-Levy.

Garfinkel, H. (1967). *Studies in ethnomethodology*. Englewood Cliffs: Prentice-Hall.

Haxaire, C., Bodénez, P., Richard, E., and Terrien, K. (2003). *Gestion différencielle des dépendances par les médecins généralistes (zones urbaines et rurales de Bretagne Occidentale)*. Retrieved from the OFDT website: http://bdoc.ofdt.fr/index.php?lvl=notice_display&id=20878.

Haxaire, C., Terrien, K., Bodénez, P., and Richard, E. (2005). From the doctor's psychotropic medication to the patient's remedies, or subversion of medicalization. *Antropologia Medica*, *19–20*, 79–92.

Reinert, M. (1992). *Logiciel ALCESTE pour l'analyse des données textuelles*. Version 2.0 [software]. Toulouse: Université de Toulouse Le Mirail, CNRS.

Reinert, M. (1993). Les 'mondes lexicaux' et leur 'logique' à travers l'analyse statistique d'un corpus de récits de cauchemar. *Langage et Société*, *66*, 5–39.

Wittgenstein, L. (1982). *Remarques sur le rameau d'or de Frazer*. Lausanne: L'Age d'Homme.

Part IV
NEW SUBJECTIVITIES, SOCIALITIES, AND THE MEDIA

11   New forms of sociality on the Internet

Users, advocates, and opponents of self-medication

Sylvie Fainzang

Introduction

Anyone examining new forms of sociality in the health domain today is expected to refer to the concept of 'biosociality' first proposed by Rabinow (2005), which aims to account for the grouping of people based on their common genomic characteristics. However, forms of health-related socialities exist that are not built on biological phenomena.

Indeed, though healthcare is generally associated with visiting a doctor and establishing a doctor–patient relationship, we are seeing an increase in people choosing to self-medicate in France today. People decide for themselves whether they are ill, and when and how to treat themselves. In order to make these decisions and choices, they refer to various sources in order to inform their actions: close friends and family, pharmacists, the media, and more and more frequently, the Internet, with its specialized websites or discussion forums. On these sites, diverse exchanges take place when participants share their experiences. Just as the search for therapeutic information engenders socialities, cybernetic relationships in return influence the way in which individuals treat their health problems.

A second use of the Internet consists of taking a stand—advocating for or against the practice of self-medication and the issue of over-the-counter medicines that have been made available through policy changes in the last few years. Self-medication and over-the-counter sales have thus become a subject of public debate in this new space of the Internet, where people exchange opinions on the risks, knowledge, and competence of individuals. Here, professional, political, and citizen voices express their opinions and opposing viewpoints are offered by various actors: public authorities, the pharmaceutical industry, doctors, pharmacists, and self-medicating individuals. In so doing, each adds their own subjectivity to bolster the interest groups they embody, and each acts for various therapeutic, economic, or political reasons.

The socialities that emerge through using the Internet in the context of self-medication generally take two forms:
1) Seeking: Participating in discussion forums in order to learn how to treat illness, or to exchange advice on medicinal use.

2) Advocating or opposing: Contributing to an Internet-based discussion, launched for example by a consumer magazine or health website, in order to give an opinion on the practice of self-medication and direct access to medicines.

What distinguishes and what unites these two forms? What are the diverse new socialities involved, and what are the common issues at stake in these new forms of sociality? My analysis shows that these two types of exchange, and the resulting new forms of sociality, are divided into practical and theoretical parts, where the main issue is the enactment of autonomy

To inform and be informed

Since patient use of medical websites, forums, and discussion lists has today come to symbolize the democratization of knowledge, more and more social scientists have taken an interest in the subject (Hardey, 1999; Akrich and Méadel, 2004). Thoer et al. (2008) emphasize, following Giddens (1991), that the availability of health-related information on the Internet allows laypeople to reappropriate knowledge; as a tool, this helps to free patients from biomedical domination because it enables the empowerment of individuals regarding their health. This echoes Hardey (1999) who notes that the Internet is the site of a new struggle over expertise in health, transforming the relationship between health professionals and their clients, which is a worrying transformation for health professionals in that they risk losing their role as the exclusive holders of expert knowledge.

Clearly, the information found on the Internet does not only come from professional sites. Information distributed by specialists on sites for the general public, whether approved by health institutions or not, is collected together with information based on the experiences of others who contribute to discussion forums. The two are sometimes mixed in accounts given by patients. From this point of view, 'searching the Internet' combines expert knowledge and lay opinions (to use the terminology favoured by sociologists), in order to compare differing points of view, in other words, to mobilize academic or professional knowledge as well as knowledge from personal experience. The phrase 'consulting the Internet' thus covers heterogeneous practices, since visiting a public forum and looking at a professional site are different social practices.

Consulting the Internet to answer health questions has led to serious concerns among those who believe that the proliferation of non-validated information constitutes a danger for individuals. While some are troubled by the lack of controls over Internet content, Akrich and Meadel (2009) note that laypeople possess a high degree of expertise. Some people become true experts on their illness and invest considerable energy reading and commenting on the Internet for the benefit of others. In this respect, studies have shown that patients using the Internet are more informed than doctors think, since they are assisted by more experienced patients (Wyatt et al., 2004), and that they are capable of making reasonable assertions on medical matters (Nettleton et al., 2005).

The building of cybernetic relationships in the health domain is, for the most part, the result of a desire to collect personal accounts concerning the efficacy of a medicine and its associated risks. In the context of self-medication, people make medicinal choices not only based on their own experience or the experiences of family and friends, but on those of anonymous Internet users. Although self-medication implies personal choice, individuals are never alone, nor are they totally independent—they are subject to a thousand influences, from those around them as well as the larger society. The aim is to benefit from the experience of other people on the Internet, despite their anonymity, concerning the efficacy of a medicine, the level of satisfaction, or a medicine's potential side effects. People turn to discussion forums in particular when they are confronted with a symptom they do not recognize, in order to identify its etiology and its seriousness. For example, Mme F. experienced a very uncomfortable sensation when eating and drinking—a bitter taste filled her mouth as soon as she consumed anything. The feeling was so troublesome that she began to think it was pathological. She considered taking antihistamines to control what she thought was an allergy, and went on an Internet discussion forum where she learned from various accounts that this disagreeable sensation could be caused by the consumption of a variety of pine nut from China—a type of pine nut that she had indeed eaten the day before—and that the symptom generally disappeared of its own accord after around a week. This information saved her from resorting to medical treatment.

Although forums are primarily consulted in order to gain information on specific medicines and illnesses, a secondary benefit of this strategy is that socialities are established through placing trust in the knowledge and experience of others. In web forums, individuals discuss precautions to be taken, conditions to adhere to in order to guarantee a medicine is innocuous, and the risks of interactions between medicines. One person thus queried: 'Is it possible to take Doliprane at the same time as Zelitrex? I have herpes on my lip which is very painful and a splitting migraine.

I am desperate, please reply.' People may prefer searching for opinions on forums over asking a pharmacist, out of embarrassment (a pharmacy does not lend itself to intimate talk about the body), for convenience (the advice arrives quicker), or simply to gain several points of view. Likewise, opinions gathered in one's social environment (family, friends, colleagues) can complement or compete with opinions gathered on the Internet.

Visiting these forums does not necessarily mean active participation. Visitors may simply be hoping to find out about a problem or a medicine from a discussion in which they do not actively participate or express an opinion, although they may identify with those who are actively participating. Even if there is no exchange of points of view to speak of, a sociality is nevertheless established. This situation is comparable to a group of people in which some listen without speaking—the speakers know they will be heard (or, in the case of the Internet, read) by the others. In other cases, exchanges are established, sometimes in an occasional manner, sometimes repeatedly, when participants express themselves several times and turn their exchanges with others into real conversations that double up as an exchange of services.

The use of forums thus establishes new forms of sociality since the criteria at the base of ordinary socialities are modified because of the anonymity of participants. Someone can contribute to a discussion by revealing a private problem affecting their body (for example, haemorrhoids, erectile dysfunction, or female hirsutism), whereas in ordinary socialities, embarrassment and the rules of social acceptability would stop them from doing so. Because participation in these forums is characterized by anonymity, exchanges can unfold between people of different ages concerning gynaecological, urological, and sexual problems; while within the context of ordinary relationships in social life, an elderly person would not generally reveal information concerning his or her body to a young person. This form of sociality is oblivious to gender, age, and to a certain extent, social background. The social and sociodemographic variables that organize and constrain ordinary forms of sociality on a subject as intimate as the body and its malfunctions are abandoned in this anonymous context. This liberates discussions that would normally be withheld, even sometimes, as we have seen, from pharmacists or doctors.

Forms of sociality created by searching for information on an illness and treatment, or the desire to transmit knowledge and experience, are both the constituents and the secondary consequences of these exchanges. It is remarkable that such exchanges are peppered with polite phrases identical to those governing forms of sociality observable in everyday life, such as 'please', 'you're welcome', and 'thank you'. For example, one might pose a question on a forum like this: 'Hello everyone, here is my problem: Do you think that this medicine could cause such side effects? Thank you everyone for your help! Have a good day!' or, 'Hi all, I'd like to thank you all for being able to discuss this delicate subject so openly.' Expressions of empathy such as *'Bon courage'* or 'Good luck' are common, as are phrases aiming to comfort someone showing distress when writing about their illness: 'You're not alone', or 'Hang in there'. Anger can be expressed as well, as seen in the response by a person who was reminded that 'tobacco is harmful to the arteries', who replied: 'What a stupid comment!' He came back to the site a month and a half later to write: 'Yes, I got a bit carried away, but the person replying to me was convinced I had an old person's illness, atherosclerosis, but I am only 26!' A forum visitor can also attract disapproval from the people to whom he/she reveals his problem. In one instance, someone replied, 'What do you expect us to say? You tell us how stupid you were and [...] you want some encouragement perhaps? Pffff... Words can't express... Only humans could be so stupid!'

Participants can also judge themselves, having revealed their carelessness:

> I don't know if you remember, I have already had to deal with this type of problem: 'a double dose this evening'. Well, I made the same stupid mistake this evening. Really bloody stupid! Last time I had this problem, I remember feeling strangely tired, shaking hands and body... a really bad thing I did there!! So yes, I wanted to ask you what you think the consequences could be. Does this sort of problem never happen to you? Good night all.

The obvious distress led to an encouraging reply posted the next day: 'How are you feeling this morning? I hope your night wasn't too disturbed.'

Finally, there are also humorous exchanges and interactions demonstrating the shared amusement of both participants. Some punctuate their posts with 'lol', or use emoticons expressing laughter, winks, etc. This form of sociality thus shares with ordinary socialities the expression of emotion (politeness, sympathy, antipathy, complicity, mockery, anger, encouragement), peppered with words of humour, jokes, and sometimes teasing, disapproval, even blame, just like relationships forum participants might have with their family, friends, and colleagues.

Taking a stance

The tendency for individuals to develop social connections based on the subject of self-medication can also be found in the context of the public debate on self-medication and the issue of direct access to medicines to which it is connected today. On 30 June 2008, the French Ministry of Health issued a decree authorizing a certain number of medicines to be sold over the counter in France. This has given rise to lively debates concerning access to medicine without a medical prescription, and direct access to medicines sold over the counter in pharmacies. The debate becomes even more heated when the question of over-the-counter drugs is thrown together with the issue of distribution, including the efforts of supermarkets to challenge the current monopoly of pharmacies on these goods.

I will not examine here the stances and arguments of all the groups of actors involved (public authorities, the pharmaceutical industry, doctors, pharmacists, and self-medicating individuals), as they are expressed in the public sphere. This was the focus of another study whose objective was to understand these actors' cognitive, symbolic, and ideological motivations in order to define their governing values and their underlying logic (Fainzang, 2012). I will limit my discussion to the points of view expressed in online discussions hosted by the magazine *60 millions de consommateurs* concerning open access to medicines, in which both pharmacists and laypeople participated. Competence and risk are two of the major issues discussed in these exchanges on self-medication and over-the-counter access.

Opinions expressed by pharmacists cover three aspects of the controversy. They include a mix of opinions hostile either to the concept of self-medication or to the practice of selling medicine over the counter or in supermarkets. Opinions hostile to the concept of self-medication are most often justified by evoking the danger it presents: 'It is in the USA that there are the most cases of hospitalization because of self-medication. No medicine is harmless! They are all dangerous!' one pharmacist declares. Others accept the idea of self-medication but do not agree that medicines should be available over the counter, even for cases deemed 'benign'. One pharmacist wrote: 'It is unacceptable that harmful substances are for sale over the counter', and she uses the example of the fact that 'taking aspirin when pregnant can be very serious for the fœtus'. Another commenter agrees, remarking that 'a sore throat and a headache can be the first signs of scarlet fever', and that in order to 'avoid complications, the correct treatment' must be taken 'as soon as the symptoms arise, symptoms that require seriousinvestigation'..

While some pharmacists approve of self-medication, they nevertheless stress loudly and clearly the importance of their role in providing advice, which potentially implies keeping the medicine behind the counter. Their hostility to over-the-counter drugs is sometimes linked to the risks posed by their consumption. One of them, writing under the name of the group Pharmaciens en colère, emphasizes that medicine is not an everyday consumer good: 'If medicine is sold over the counter so that we can consume it at a lower price, French people will consume even more when they are already consuming too much.'

There are several underlying rationales behind the points of view expressed by the pharmacists. Some are supporting corporations or professions, some are defending consumers and denouncing the greed of supermarkets and the pharmaceutical industry, and others are speaking up for public health. These different rationales are sometimes combined together based on the risks involved in self-medication—risks inherent in what is judged to be the incompetence of patients: 'users do not know how to recognize symptoms and cannot know if they are benign or not'; 'most French people do not know the difference between aspirin and paracetamol'. The fact that people lack medical information leads some to judge the situation to be irreparable: 'The state is acting irresponsibly. We know very well that people will not read the contraindications and an accident can happen very quickly.' This point of view sometimes takes the form of lamenting that people are incapable of self-medicating correctly in spite of the information available to them: 'It is an illusion to think that people will self-medicate responsibly; how can we be sure that patients take the correct dose, at the right time, if no one is guiding them?'

Laypeople responded to these differing opinions. While the majority are in favour of self-medication, opinions are more reserved when it comes to over-the-counter access, for either therapeutic or economic reasons. In strictly economic terms, the decree also provokes disparate reactions. Some object to reduced prices, fearing this may spur people to consume more, while others like the fact that the decree forces pharmacists to make prices on the medicines transparent. Others meanwhile predict the opposite: that the price of over-the-counter medicines will actually rise.

But the crux of the debate is above all the capacity of a patient to decide whether to acquire medicine and undergo treatment without the intervention of healthcare professionals. Some warmly welcome this increased access, while still hoping to see pharmacists continuing to provide advice and fearing that supermarkets will take over the sector: 'Is it not a bit risky to buy these substances at the same time as eggs and chocolate? Supervision performed by pharmacists during sales is not just a myth, it prevents numerous medicinal accidents', one participant declares. Others agree. One worries about the consequences of selling medicine over the counter precisely because it opens the way for supermarkets to sell these products, which implies that medicine will become trivialized: 'Pills are not sweets as represented by Leclerc in its advert showing a necklace similar to the candy necklaces we used to eat as children!' But this argument is challenged by someone who points out that pharmacists sell sweets too; still others see the fact that medicines could become available in supermarkets as a positive development. Responding to pharmacists who advocate their role as advisors, some counter that such an advisory role is simply fantasy: 'Pharmacists do not intervene to warn patients when they buy medicines that are not compatible with each other.' Another consumer confirms this: 'When we go to the pharmacy, no one asks us anything more than in the supermarket; we are served, and that's it; pharmacists have become simple shopkeepers; they are there to sell and make money, that is all!'

Finally, the availability of over-the-counter drugs, in both pharmacies and supermarkets, is warmly welcomed by certain consumers who appreciate being able to choose for themselves and resented being infantilized regarding access to these medicines, as shown by these statements: 'We are capable of taking care of our little problems!' and 'Yes, we are not kids; we know what we are doing!' On the grounds that they possess sufficient competence, they affirm their desire to take their health into their own hands and their ability to be autonomous. Another disagrees: 'Recently I almost put the life of my unborn baby in danger by taking aspirin: my pharmacist stopped me, luckily, since he said it could have been fatal for my baby', showing her appreciation for pharmacist competence. The claim that individuals possess sufficient competence is confirmed by some and challenged by others.

These exchanges serve as a sounding board for individuals' to discuss their experiences and daily practices, and in so doing they develop a sociality as an actor in the domain of self-medication. The points of view expressed fulfil various functions: they aim either to reinforce cohesion or to develop a conflicting or critical relationship between groups of social actors. While pharmacists defend a corporatist position, laypeople sometimes express criticism of pharmacists' practices that they might not dare state openly in person. Here again, the exchange of points of view is liberated by anonymity, but through a different mechanism: it is not the moral dimension of ordinary sociality that disappears here, but the social and political dimensions that would normally make face-to-face criticism of the practices of healthcare professionals difficult. Overall, these cybernetic exchanges crystallize the social relationships between drug users and pharmacists on the questions of consumer competence and autonomy.

Synthesis

Several authors have taken an interest in new forms of sociality created through links established via the Internet, or what Casilli (2010) calls 'digital links', such as those facilitated by social networks. While Casilli (2010, p. 57) speaks in terms of 'virtual sociability', I prefer not to retain the term 'virtual' because it implies that this sociability only exists as a potential. In the field of cybernetics, 'virtual' refers to a simulation of reality, but here we are dealing with its actual achievement. The so-called virtual world, as a space for communication created by the global interconnection of computers within which its users navigate, is, from an anthropological point of view, a very real world, as are the practices that take place there and the relationships that are formed there.

According to Casilli (2010, p. 57), the Internet brings new forms of interaction: 'face-to-face meetings are no longer the exclusive means of interaction'. He emphasizes that we now have multiple means to communicate without having to go anywhere (through mobile telephone, email, Internet forums, etc.), and it is no longer necessary to physically meet other people (p. 122). However, Casilli shows that the body has not disappeared, far from it: the body is very much there, at the exact centre of our daily life, as the questions raised by web users over how to stay in good health reveal. The body is omnipresent and remains at the centre of individual preoccupations.

Other authors have concentrated on forms of sociality created by chronic conditions of ill health (for example, Whyte, 2009), whether they take place on the Internet or elsewhere. Rabinow (2005) coined the term 'biosociality' to account for the manner in which biological nature, as revealed and monitored by science, constitutes the foundation of social life. He thus proposed the notion of biosocialities in the context of his work on the human genome to account for groupings of people based on their common genomic particularities. To illustrate what he means by biosociality, he takes the example of the existence of neurofibromatosis groups, 'whose members meet to share their experiences, lobby for their disease, educate their children, redo their home environment and so on' (Rabinow, 2005, p. 102). As Whyte (2012) remarks, biosociality has henceforth become one of the central questions examined in social science research on chronic illness. These works outline new forms of sociality found in patient support and advocacy groups, or seen in social transformations as a result of innovations in the genomic domain (Gibbon and Novas, 2008). Ducournau and Beaudevin (2011) document biosocialities that revolve around sharing information about one's own genetics, which they dub 'Facebook genomics'. These interactions included exchanges among people who buy genetic tests on the Internet that provide information on their predispositions to certain diseases, and who begin online exchanges because of the genetic proximity suggested by their results.

Although the exchanges of questions and advice taking place on discussion forums described here are based on a pathological condition or a particular symptom and fall within the scope of new forms of sociality in the health domain, we cannot identify these exchanges as 'biosocialities', as Beaudevin (2013) stresses that these are defined as associations of people affected by the same disease. Nor can we talk here about 'biological citizenship' (Rose and Novas, 2005). On the one hand, the biosociality argument implies that social relationships are formed on the basis of a biological phenomenon or of biological characteristics. In our case, people are not necessarily experiencing a biological transformation of their body nor do they share the same illness. On the other hand, exchanges can take place regarding a bodily reality without the person necessarily experiencing it at the time of writing or experiencing it themselves, since the discussions also refer to experiences of family and friends. Furthermore, sociality developed around a shared preoccupation at a certain moment in daily life does not necessarily imply a health 'condition', as experiencing an occasional symptom cannot be considered as identical to living with a chronic illness. Finally, sociality is based on sharing a common concern for a body experience that might be but is not necessarily pathological, or a body experience that is not recognized as pathological by medical professionals (Fainzang, 2013).

The information sharing examined above is perhaps closer to the notion of 'therapeutic citizenship' as defined by Nguyen (2005), in which expert clients are incorporated into healthcare activities, with the difference that these exchanges do not involve active healing but centre instead on giving advice on health—creating what might be called 'health citizenship'. This term is more appropriate to account for what is happening in these new forms of sociality, since the exchanges are pursued in order to encourage or dissuade recourse to a treatment or a specific medicine, but neither 'seekers' nor 'advocates' are in fact incorporated into the healing activity. It is only the self-medicating person who participates in the healthcare activity, thus exercising their therapeutic citizenship. From the synthesis of therapeutic citizenship (asking for advice in order to self-administer treatment) and health citizenship (exchanging advice about health) comes 'health sociality'. In the situation where people take a stance on self-medication, it involves asserting a citizen's point of view regarding an offer of services and a therapeutic strategy, without playing a therapeutic role. The aim is thus to assert a posture, for or against self-medication, linked to a philosophical, or even political, position on the question of autonomy and user competence. This position participates in health citizenship since the key issue is to define the conditions in which it is judged reasonable or not to treat oneself alone, and to express an opinion on the validity or not of self-medication and access to over-the-counter medicines.

These diverse forms of sociality are based either on the experience of a symptom, an ailment, or a medicine—as a user—or on a personal doctrine concerning the recourse to self-medication—as an advocate or opponent. In the first configuration, they are the result of a therapeutic quest; in the second, they are the result of a quest for social recognition and the assertion of competence within the domain. In both cases, social exchanges are created on the basis of the legal, social, and physiological possibility of managing one's own body. These exchanges aim either to improve the efficacy of one's practice or to give it legitimacy; they all stem from a desire to make one's voice heard or to interact with the bodies of others. In conclusion, the forms of sociality developing among users, advocates, and opponents of self-medication in the cybernetic space, form a diptych, practical and theoretical, on the issue of autonomy: autonomy in principle versus autonomy in action.

References

Akrich, M., and Méadel, C. (2004). Problématiser la question des usages. *Sciences Sociales et Santé, 22*(1), 5–20.

Akrich, M., and Méadel, C. (2009). Internet: Intrus ou médiateur dans la relation patient/médecin? *Santé, Société et Solidarité, 2*, 87–91.

Beaudevin, C. (2013). Old diseases and contemporary crisis: Inherited blood disorders in Oman. *Anthropology & Medicine, 20*(2), 175–189.

Casilli, A.A. (2010). *Les liaisons numériques*. La couleur des idées. Paris: Le Seuil.

Ducournau, P., and Beaudevin, C. (2011). Génétique en ligne: Déterritorialisation des régulations de santé publique et formes de développement commercial. *Anthropologie et Santé, 3*. Retrieved from http://anthropologiesante.revues.org/777.

Fainzang, S. (2012). *L'automédication ou les mirages de l'autonomie*. Paris: Presses Universitaires de France.

Fainzang, S. (2013). The other side of medicalization: Self-medicalization and self-medication. *Culture, Medicine, and Psychiatry, 37*(3), 488–504.

Gibbon, S., and Novas, C. (2008). *Biosocialities, genetics and the social sciences: Making biologies and identities.* London: Routledge.

Giddens, A. (1991). *Modernity and self-identity.* Cambridge: Polity Press.

Hardey, M. (1999). Doctor in the house: The Internet as a source of lay health knowledge and the challenge to expertise. *Sociology of Health and Illness, 21*(6), 820–835.

Nettleton, S., Burrows, R., and O'Malley, L. (2005). The mundane realities of the everyday lay use of the Internet for health and their consequences for media convergence. *Sociology of Health and Illness, 27*(7), 972–992.

Nguyen, V.-K. (2005). Antiretroviral globalism, biopolitics, and therapeutic citizenship. In A. Ong and S.J. Collier, eds., *Global assemblages: Technology, politics, and ethics as anthropological problems* (pp. 124–144). Malden: Blackwell.

Rabinow, P. (2005). Artificiality and enlightenment: From sociobiology to biosociality. In J.X. Inda, ed., *Anthropologies of modernity: Foucault, governmentality and life politics* (pp. 179–193). Oxford: Blackwell.

Rose, N., and Novas, C. (2005). Biological citizenship. In A. Ong and S.J. Collier, eds., *Global assemblages: Technology, politics, and ethics as anthropological problems* (pp. 439–463). Malden: Blackwell.

Thoer, C., Pierret, J., and Lévy, J.J. (2008). Quelques réflexions sur des pratiques d'utilisation des médicaments hors cadre medical. *Drogues, santé et société, 7*(1), 19–54.

Whyte, S.R. (2009). Health identities and subjectivities: The ethnographic challenge. *Medical Anthropology Quarterly, 23*(1), 6–15.

Whyte, S.R. (2012). Chronicity and control: Framing noncommunicable diseases in Africa. *Anthropology & Medicine, 19*(1), 63–74.

Wyatt, S., Henwood, F., Hart, A., and Platzer, H. (2004). L'extension des territoires du patient: Internet et santé au quotidian. *Sciences Sociales et Santé, 22*(1), 45–68.

12 'The Internet saved my life'

Overcoming isolation among the homebound chronically ill

Lina Masana

Introduction

Some of the constraints imposed by chronic illness prevent people from having what is understood as a 'normal life' that includes working outside the home and maintaining regular social relationships. Some chronically ill people are obliged to spend all day at home, often alone, with few opportunities to meet other people, converse, or express their feelings. They feel isolated and alone. Fortunately, the Internet[1] has changed this situation for many, creating new forms of sociality.

Three decades ago, virtual social relationships in cyberspace[2] would have been inconceivable; today, we take them for granted. As a window to the outside world, the Internet has helped many homebound, chronically ill people overcome social isolation.[3] Participation in patients' online communities, forums, self-help groups, blogs, and other health-related web pages is becoming an important source of moral, emotional, and social support[4] because it enables the sharing of common experiences and interests (Burrows et al., 2000; Josefsson, 2005; Nettleton et al., 2002). Moreover, the Internet has created conditions for the emergence of new forms of care (Atkinson and Ayers, 2010; Burrows et al., 2000)—both *caring for* and *caring about*—not only among the chronically ill but also between sick and healthy people.

1   Also referred to as the 'Net'.
2   The notions of *virtual relationships, virtual social life*, and *online relationships* are understood here as forms of social interaction in a virtual environment, using computer-mediated practices (also called *online practices*) that are related to the concept of *virtual communities* (see Hine, 2004; Miller and Slater, 2000; Rheingold, 1996; Woolgar, 2010). Virtual life should not be understood as opposed to 'real' life, but as part of it, because both are parallel and simultaneous dimensions of people's lives (Wilson and Peterson, 2002; Woolgar, 2002).
3   While this contribution's primary focus is on the social constraints of being homebound, the creation of virtual relationships on the Internet is not exclusive to those who are chronically ill and homebound, or even to those who are ill in any way.
4   Support is given within these three dimensions—moral, emotional and social—and not simply one because they are often closely related. Elsewhere I have explored the significance of this multidimensional support in relation to chronic illness (see Masana, 2010).

Social relations are especially important in times of illness and other adversities. Online forms of sociality among the ill and homebound have received little attention because the ethnographic gaze usually focuses instead on face-to-face relationships. Virtual sociality challenges us to re-think our concepts of 'data' and our methodological approaches to 'the field' (Hookway, 2008; Hine, 2004, 2005, 2007; Jacobson, 1999; Mann and Stewart, 2000; Murthy, 2012; Turkle, 1995; Wilson and Peterson, 2002; Sixsmith and Murray, 2001). The aim of this contribution is to show how the Internet has partly helped to overcome the isolation and loneliness that accompany some chronic illnesses, and how it enables new types of socialities and new care practices at a distance.

Real people, *virtual* lives

The data reported here are drawn from my doctoral research on the experi-ence and management of chronic illness in Catalonia, Spain, and focuses on 20 adults between 30 and 50 years old, a subset of my total sample. The narratives quoted in this chapter come from two different sources: in-depth personal interviews conducted between 2009 and 2011 at the homes of chronically ill people, and four months of weekly observation in 2010 in a therapeutic group at the chronic pain unit of a prominent regional hospital in Catalonia in 2010. All participants in the study live in urban areas or in villages close to urban centres, and, with few exceptions, have a computer with an Internet connection, which they use daily for different purposes. Some are now working part-time or full-time, or have some kind of activ-ity outside the home, but had been homebound during certain phases of their illnesses. The others are on long-term sick leave or have some kind of permanent disability pension, and are thus indefinitely homebound. None of the participants are *digital natives*,[5] but those with computers and the Internet use it for social relations, entertainment, and health-related issues. Those who do not have a computer or use the Internet consider themselves 'too old for that', and unable to learn the necessary skills to enter, as one of them put it, this 'difficult and strange world'.

---

5   This term is used to identify those born during or after the general introduction of digital technology and to suggest they began using and interacting with digital technology at an early age.

Illness, the Internet, and social life

We can observe two main tendencies in studies of lay use of the Internet in relation to health and illness. First, most studies tend to analyse the e-health phenomenon, that is, use of the Internet as a source of health information for laypersons (Hardey, 1999, 2002; Nettleton et al., 2004, 2005).[6] These practices include acquiring knowledge about one's disease, symptoms, or treatment; seeking medical and lay advice; formulating a self-diagnosis or looking for a medical diagnosis; and attaining a level of 'expertise' in self-medication, among others. These practices focus on the professional–patient relationship and on the medical condition—the disease—and at issue are questions of knowledge, expertise, empowerment, and autonomy.

Second, other studies (Flinkfeldt, 2011; Josefsson, 2005; Loader et al., 2002; Nettleton et al., 2002) have examined the virtual social lives of the chronically ill as new forms of care and social support made possible by the Internet. Personal accounts of illness through blogs, patients' online communities, self-help groups and forums, Facebook, and Twitter allow us to study relationships between the healthy and the sick and among the sick. These uses of the Internet that pertain to the personal and social experience of illness, not merely the disease, are the focus of this study.[7]

Before the Internet age, receiving visits at home or talking on the phone was the primary way for a homebound chronically ill person to maintain social relationships beyond the domestic unit. While the Internet has opened a window for potential new socialities, it does not, however, exclude previous forms of social interaction (Woolgar, 2002). Despite widespread use of the Internet, some people do not have an Internet connection or a computer, or the skills to use either.[8] Some may have all three, but decide

6   See also Fainzang in this volume.

7   Content and interactional style in patients' online communities, self-help groups, and forums vary considerably according to cultural context. For instance, some of my study participants distinguish between the 'style' of some Spanish websites versus those in the United States. They valued US sites positively because they contain 'more disease-related information', although the volume of information may sometimes be overwhelming. Personal accounts of illness on US sites were also seen as 'too exaggerated and dramatic'. Similarly, Nettleton et al. (2005), in a UK-based study, found that some British participants avoided 'American stuff' because they considered it 'too dramatic'. Further research attentive to culturally specific Internet 'styles' would illuminate the dynamics of the use of these websites by the chronically ill. This chapter focuses not on Catalan-specific uses of the Internet for social relationships, but on common practices among the chronically ill for overcoming isolation and loneliness.

8   Accessibility and ability, among other structural and social context factors, are the main reasons for the use (or not) of the Internet (Woolgar, 2002).

not to use the Internet for health- or illness-related purposes. Using the Internet may therefore be a personal choice for some, while for others it may be their only option. How has the Internet changed or affected the lives of the chronically ill and homebound? How are these new forms of sociality perceived by those who are homebound and chronically ill?

Montse, a woman in her 40s suffering from severely debilitating fibromyalgia, was homebound on long-term sick leave. Despite her illness, she was able to spend hours in front of the computer, and was enthusiastic about her time there:

> Oh, the Internet saved my life! I spend a lot of hours every day in front of the computer [smiling enthusiastically]. I read all the posts in the forum, I answer many of them, I chat with friends, we send each other pictures, songs, or whatever. It's my only way not to be alone. When I am *there* [on the Internet] I feel alive, I almost forget about my pain. Anyway, I can't do other things. What I should do? Lie in bed all day long? That would kill me. And yes, it is painful and tiring to spend so many hours sitting in a chair in front of the screen, but at least *there* I have a life, I have friends, we talk, I am not alone *there*. (Emphasis added)

When Montse says that the Internet saved her life, she is not talking about relief for her medical condition; she is talking about feeling alive, being 'in the world' and connected to others who support her and help her to manage the effects of the illness on her life, including the possibility of social death, as implied in her reference to a bed-bound life without social interaction. The Internet offers virtual social life and interaction that provides new forms of moral, emotional, and social support (Nettleton et al., 2002), and alternative caring practices—both caring *for* and caring *about* (Atkinson and Ayers, 2010; Burrows et al., 2000)—that 'save' not the body but the souls of those who are homebound and chronically ill.

Chronically ill on the Net: Navigating or participating?

There are two main forms of engagement with the Internet[9]: *to use it* or *to be in it*, or, in other words, *navigating* or *participating*. The first option consists of navigating through web pages searching for disease-related information or reading personal accounts of illness experiences posted on blogs, chat

9   See Nettleton et al. (2004) for a further description of 'health e-types'.

rooms, or forums, without interacting in any way with others. The second implies interaction: responding to others' posts and participating (more or less actively) in online communities, chats, or forums. Although I am more interested here in participatory and interactive uses of the Internet, in my research I observed that even those who limit themselves to navigating without participating may also feel helped by reading others' illness accounts. Laura, for example, a 46-year-old woman suffering from four invisible chronic conditions that she has not disclosed to many of her co-workers or friends, and who jealously guards her privacy and anonymity, is reluctant to participate or to 'show' herself (as she says) on the Internet, but she does look at it sometimes and read what other chronically ill people write:

> I don't write anything and don't get in touch with anybody. No. I just read. But by reading, I see others that have a similar situation to mine, and *it helps* me to understand that *I am not the only one*. You know, sometimes you feel like you are the only miserable one suffering in the world. And that's not true. Many others suffer like you. It is good to know, because *you feel less alone*. (Emphasis added)

While the Internet allows anonymity, many people share a lot of personal and private information about themselves on the Internet. In some cases they create online nicknames in order not to be recognized, but others state clearly who they are, where they live, and other personal data. Although Laura could participate online in an anonymous way, she chose not to do it; for her, 'just reading' had already made a positive impact by allowing her to see that she is not alone, and that knowledge helped her bear her own suffering.

Nevertheless, 'just reading' can also turn into a depressing, frightening, or anxiety-provoking experience for some of the already vulnerable chronic illness sufferers. When I asked Mariona about her relationship with patients' online associations for her condition, she answered:

> I know that there is one [patients' association for her condition] on the Internet, but I started to read it once, and I saw people who were even worse off than me, and you know, that got me down. No, it's too depressing. You read that and it brings you to your knees—and you say 'I already know all this, and I don't need to read any more about it.'

Mariona's account shows us a phenomenon described by Goffman (1995) as a 'circle of lament'—also present in some self-help groups and patients' associations offline—that may have a counterproductive effect on those who were initially looking for relief and support, but come away from the encounter with additional burdens and worries. What can be a good, useful, and supportive experience for some may be bad, useless, or even harmful for others, which may lead some chronically ill people to choose not to seek out such sites.

Participating actively on the Internet enables chronically ill people to share their illness experience with others who suffer from the same disease or a similar situation (Atkinson and Ayers, 2010; Hardey, 2002). Through sharing 'the story of a common problem' (Canals, 2002, 2003; Silverman, 1980), those who do choose to participate actively are able to develop and maintain social relationships and form part of a community[10] (Hardey, 2002) that keeps them anchored in 'the world', as my study participants expressed it, even if they are unable to leave the house. Interacting with one's peers implies better mutual understanding of the adversity of one another's situations (Goffman, 1995). Some chronically ill people feel more comfortable sharing their lives with others in similar situations because they know in advance that they will not be judged, mistreated, disbelieved, or delegitimized by others. Participating in such forums, chats, or other types of online communities fosters a sense of belonging, which is in turn essentially linked to moral, emotional, and social support. As Montse says:

> We all know what it is. We don't judge, we support each other. One day I feel bad and another member cheers me up. And maybe another day that other person feels miserable and I can help her to deal with it. At least we share the same thing, we all know what we are talking about. We don't need to hide, or pretend, or fake anything. We are just [as] we are, ill people.

Virtual social relationships develop not only among the ill, but between the sick and the healthy as well. Mariona, who is now 36, made new healthy friends through the Internet. She was born with a congenital cardiopathy and has suffered from pulmonary hypertension since the age of 28, when her condition forced her to stop working outside the home. In the beginning

---

10   For a discussion of the concept of community in mutual support groups, see Canals (1998). On virtual communities, see Burrows et al. (2002); Castells (2001); Josefsson (2005); Rheingold (1996).

she lost some friends[11] because she was unable to take part in their regular social activities, and this made her even less inclined to leave the house. When I asked about her social life, she explained how she managed to rebuild it after three years of homebound isolation, ending nearly in tears:

> We created a group of friends on the Internet, through the chat. It was a very good [experience] for me, because I could escape from being shut in here [at home]. We have lunch and do other things together, and now I can enjoy life again like other [healthy young] people. This did me a lot of good, because I had spent three years very closed in [on] myself, because, you know, I spent all my time worrying about my illness, and when you talk to other people you don't know what else to talk about, it's just the illness and, you know, I was so closed off.

Online rules for virtual relationships: Unexpected consequences, negative outcomes

While the Internet has a positive impact on the lives of many chronically ill people, others have had negative experiences. As in everyday face-to-face interaction, online communities and virtual relationships operate according to rules that are both explicit and implicit. Disrespectful and offensive language is explicitly prohibited, and other implicit rules, grounded in reciprocity (Mauss, 1971) as a central value, are demanded. This involves regular communication: posting often, responding to others' posts, asking and answering questions, and sharing intimate details of one's personal experience—all in all, the quid pro quo rule. Clara once tried to get involved in an online forum of people suffering from fibromyalgia and chronic fatigue syndrome recommended by some members of a biweekly therapy group she was attending. She could not, however, keep up with all the news, posts, and chats because she often felt too unwell to spend the necessary time sitting in front of the screen reading and responding to others' posts and writing her own. Surprisingly for her, these peers whom she assumed would be more understanding and supportive complained about her online behaviour:

> Every time I went to the therapy group, if I hadn't been very active and didn't participate enough [online], they complained and said, 'Ah, you

---

11   Losing friends can be one of the unpleasant negative outcomes of living with a chronic illness (see Frank, 1991; Kleinman, 1988).

don't show up', 'Oh, you aren't answering any messages', 'Oh, you never write anything about yourself', 'You're always off', 'You don't care', and so on. They made me feel so bad with their complaints! I couldn't do otherwise, I can't spend as many hours at the computer as they do, reading and reading and reading, and answering, answering, answering. No, I couldn't and I can't. THEY should understand, but some don't. So I quit. (Capital letters added to emphasize the tone and intensity of the oral account)

One of the main characteristics of virtual interaction is its temporal structure: it allows for asynchronous as well as synchronous communication, which is an important feature for the chronically ill, because it allows them to participate whenever they feel well enough to do so, at their convenience. Some people may not be able to stay on top of things all the time—if at all—and one might expect other people with chronic illnesses to be more accepting of this. Complaints such as those Clara received from her peers are related to the perception that she had broken the implicit rules of reciprocity. Because she did not write, respond, participate, or communicate with the expected frequency or in expected ways, she disappointed the others. In Clara's own words, she had broken the unspoken rule: 'Don't expect me to share my life with you if you are not willing to share yours with me, or if you are not going to say anything in return.' Clara's unpleasant experience was not unusual; other study participants recounted similar experiences. Negative responses from peers can lead some chronically ill to withdraw from engaging in these online communities.

Sharing and caring

Sharing information about 'the story of my illness' (Hardey, 2002) is generally intended to 'help others' in a similar difficult situation: to learn more about the disease; to show people how others manage the situation; to express support; to give advice; to cheer people up; and, of utmost importance, to let others know that 'you are not alone'. The latter is a key and often-repeated message, since those who are aware of the social constraints of illness know firsthand that social isolation and loneliness are among the biggest fears of the homebound chronically ill. Sharing one's life with others in an empathic way—'I know what you've been through'—generates a sense of belonging and shows that others *care about* you. As Montse says, 'We do care, we care about the others. And we take care of each other. Feeling supported allows us to deal with it [the illness] better, because not feeling alone is very important.'

Another characteristic of online social interactions is its *expressiveness*. Along with comforting words, jokes, and other forms of humour intended to lift people's spirits, participants also share 'emoticons': virtual smiles, winks, hugs, kisses, flowers, suns, and so on. All these displays of affection, which I understand as caring practices that provide moral, emotional, and social support, bring people together and create a sense of closeness, belonging, friendship, and companionship. The Internet removes physical boundaries and enables *caring at a distance* from one's home: being *there* [online] enables being in the *world*, having a social presence, caring for others and being cared for, which is important for those who are homebound and physically isolated.

As I have argued elsewhere (Masana, 2010), we tend to understand care practices as limited to functional activities or tasks. My data show that the sharing of information and experience on the Internet also constitutes a form of caring both for and about others, even when this is not the explicit intention. *Human understanding* in itself is a form of support (Josefsson, 2005).

Final considerations

Virtual social relationships create new forms of socialities that allow homebound chronically ill people to partly overcome isolation and loneliness. People engaged in these online illness communities play an active and reciprocal role in caring practices: they care for/about others just as others care for/about them. Proof of this is the fact that most illness-related web pages, blogs, and forums are initiated and promoted by people with those illnesses, because they want to help, inform, advise, and support others facing similarly adverse conditions (Atkinson and Ayers, 2010; Burrows et al., 2000; Flinkfeldt, 2011; Hardey, 2002; Josefsson, 2005; Loader et al., 2002).

This does not, however, mean that chronically ill people spend all day in virtual contact only with others like themselves. They may also have active virtual social lives through Facebook, Twitter, and other social networks not specifically related to health and illness. The Internet allows homebound chronically ill people to build relationships not only with other chronically ill people, but also with healthy ones, and in this way it makes it possible for them to remain connected to others.

The virtual and the 'real' are not mutually exclusive dimensions of social life (Wilson and Peterson, 2002; Woolgar, 2002). People can 'play' in both at the same time. Moreover, all people (healthy or sick) can combine face-to-face relationships with virtual ones, and in some cases they may meet in person those whom they get to know through the Internet. The difference, however, is that for people whose lives are constrained by chronic illnesses severe enough to keep them from leaving their homes or even receiving visits, virtual social life may be the only option available.[12] For these people, the Internet becomes an important window to the outside world that overcomes physical boundaries, evidenced in statements like these: 'It's like going out [from home] and meeting other people [chronically ill or healthy]', and 'It's like a meeting place for us [other people with chronic illness]'.

Although still underrepresented in the literature, virtual relationships and communities constitute a new ethnographic field (Armstrong et al., 2012; Capogrossi et al., 2015; Kozinets, 2010; Mudry and Strong, 2013; O'Brien and Clark, 2012; Paechter, 2013; Rodriquez, 2013).[13] The analysis of narratives from the Internet—so-called virtual ethnography or netnography—still encounters some resistance because it challenges our well-established ethnographic methods: face-to-face interviews and direct observation (Hine, 2004; Turkle, 1995), raises new ethical concerns (Hookway, 2008; Jacobson, 1999; Paechter, 2013; Sixsmith and Murray, 2001; Wilson and Peterson, 2002), and exposes the limitations of the traditional concept of 'the field' that contrasts with 'home' and is predicated on the 'naturalization of cultural difference as inhering in different geographical locales' (Gupta and Ferguson, 1997, p. 8). Nevertheless, this field cannot be ignored and further research—for example, on culture-specific or gendered uses of the Internet—is needed to build up ethnographic data that will allow us to gain insight into this relatively new form of social interaction among the chronically ill.

Acknowledgements

I am grateful to the participants of the seventh Medical Anthropology at Home conference held in Driebergen, the Netherlands (2012), and

---

12   Severe cases of multiple chemical sensitivities would be an example of this, as described in the blog created by a young Spanish woman, Eva Caballé, who must live completely isolated from the outside world (see http://nofun-eva.blogspot.com/p/sobre-mi.html, last accessed 22 May 2012).

13   Please note that this chapter was written in early 2012, and that while a few more publications have appeared since, more are needed.

particularly Sylvie Fainzang and Bernhard Hadolt for their constructive comments on an earlier draft of this paper and suggestions for improving it.

Funding

This research was conducted thanks to a pre-doctoral fellowship for junior researchers (2008–2011) supported by the Commission for Universities and Research of the Department of Innovation, Universities and Enterprise of the Generalitat de Catalunya, and the European Social Fund. Additional support came from a later mobility grant (2012) from the Secretariat for Universities and Research and the Department of Economy and Knowledge of the Generalitat de Catalunya (the Catalan government of the autonomous community of Catalonia, Spain).

References

Armstrong, N., Koteyko, N., and Powell, J. (2012). 'Oh dear, should I really be saying that on here?' Issues of identity and authority in an online diabetes community. *Health*, *16*(4), 347–365.

Atkinson, S., and Ayers, A. (2010). The potential of the Internet for alternative caring practices for health. *Anthropology and Medicine*, *17*(1), 75–86.

Burrows, R., Nettleton, S., Pleace, N., Loader, B., and Muncer, S. (2000). Virtual community care? Social policy and the emergence of computer mediated social support. *Information, Communication & Society*, *3*(1), 95–121.

Canals, J. (1998). La reconstrucción imaginaria de la comunidad: Consideraciones sobre un tópico del reformismo sanitario. *Trabajo Social y Salud*, *29*, 267–278.

Canals, J. (2002). *El regreso de la reciprocidad: Grupos de ayuda mutua y asociaciones de personas afectadas en la crisis del Estado del Bienestar* [The return of reciprocity: Mutual help groups and associations of affected persons in the welfare state crisis]. Unpublished doctoral dissertation. Departament d'Antropologia, Filosofia i Treball Social, Universitat Rovira i Virgili, Tarragona, Spain.

Canals, J. (2003). Grupos de ayuda mutua y asociaciones de personas afectadas: Reciprocidades, identidades y dependencias [Mutual help groups and patient support associations: Reciprocity, identity and dependency]. *Cuadernos de Psiquiatría Comunitaria*, *3*(1), 71–81.

Capogrossi, M.L., Magallanes M.L., and Soraire, F. (2015) Los desafíos de Facebook: Apuntes para el abordaje de las redes sociales como fuente. *Antropologia Experimental*, *15*(4), 47–63.

Castells, M. (2001). *La galàxia internet*. Barcelona: Plaza and Janés.

Flinkfeldt, M. (2011). Filling one's days: Managing sick leave legitimacy in an online forum. *Sociology of Health & Illness*, *33*(5), 761–776.

Frank, A.W. (1991). *At the will of the body: Reflections on illness*. Boston: Houghton Mifflin.

Goffman, E. (1995) *Estigma: La identidad deteriorada* [Stigma: Notes on the management of spoiled identity]. L. Guinsberg, trans. Buenos Aires: Amorrortu. (Original work published in 1963.)

Gupta, A., and Ferguson, J. (1997). Discipline and practice: 'The field' as site, method and location in anthropology. In A. Gupta and J. Ferguson, eds., *Anthropological locations: Boundaries and grounds of a field science* (pp. 1–46). Berkeley: University of California Press.

Hardey, M. (1999). Doctor in the house: The Internet as a source of lay health knowledge and the challenge to expertise. *Sociology of Health & Illness*, 21(6), 820–835.

Hardey, M. (2002). 'The story of my illness': Personal accounts of illness on the Internet. *Health*, 6(1), 31–46.

Hine, C. (2004). *Etnografía virtual* [Virtual ethnography]. Barcelona: UOC. (Original work published in 2000.)

Hine, C. (2005). *Virtual methods: Issues in social research on the Internet.* Oxford: Berg.

Hine, C. (2007). Multi-sited ethnography as a middle range methodology for contemporary STS. *Science, Technology, & Human Values*, 32(6), 652–671.

Hookway, N. (2008). 'Entering the blogosphere': Some strategies for using blogs in social research. *Qualitative Research*, 8(1), 91–113.

Jacobson, D. (1999). Doing research in cyberspace. *Field Methods*, 11(2), 127–145.

Josefsson, U. (2005). Coping with illness online: The case of patients' online communities. *The Information Society*, 21, 143–153.

Kleinman, A. (1988). *The illness narratives: Suffering, healing and the human condition.* New York: Basic Books.

Kozinets, R.V. (2010). *Netnography: Doing ethnographic research online.* Los Angeles, CA: Sage.

Loader, B., Muncer, S., Burrows, R., Pleace, N., and Nettleton, S. (2002). Medicine on the line? Computer-mediated social support and advice for people with diabetes. *International Journal of Social Welfare*, 11, 53–65.

Mann, C., and Stewart, F. (2000). *Internet communication and qualitative research: A handbook for researching online.* London: Sage.

Masana, L. (2010). Self-care and management of adults with chronic illness and dependency: The Spanish case in the context of the new dependency law. In S. Fainzang, H.E. Hem, and M.B. Risor, eds., *The taste for knowledge: Medical anthropology facing medical realities* (pp. 199–218). Aarhus: Aarhus University Press.

Mauss, M. (1971). Ensayo sobre los dones: Motivo y forma del cambio en las sociedades primitivas. In G. Gurvitch, ed., *Sociología y Antropología*, 2nd ed. (pp. 153–263). Madrid: Tecnos. (Original work published in 1923–1924.)

Miller, D., and Slater, D. (2000). *The Internet: An ethnographic approach.* Oxford: Berg.

Mudry, T.E., and Strong, T. (2013). Doing recovery online. *Qualitative Health Research* 23(3), 313–325.

Murthy, D. (2012). Digital ethnography: An examination of the use of new technologies for social research. *Sociology*, 42(5), 837–855.

Nettleton, S., Burrows, R., and O'Malley, L. (2005). The mundane realities of the everyday lay use of the Internet for health, and their consequences for media convergence. *Sociology of Health & Illness*, 27(7), 972–992.

Nettleton, S., Burrows, R., O'Malley, L., and Watt, I. (2004). Health e-types? An analysis of the everyday use of the Internet for health. *Information, Communication & Society*, 7(4), 531–553.

Nettleton, S., Pleace, N., Burrows, R., Muncer, S., and Loader, B. (2002). The reality of virtual social support. In S. Woolgar, ed., *Virtual society? Technology, cyberole, reality* (pp. 176–188). Oxford: Oxford University Press.

O'Brien, M.R., and Clark, D. (2012). Unsolicited written narratives as a methodological genre in terminal illness: Challenges and limitations. *Qualitative Health Research*, 22, 274–284.

Paechter, C. (2013). Researching sensitive issues online: Implications of a hybrid insider/outsider position in a retrospective ethnographic study. *Qualitative Research* 13(1), 171–186.

Rheingold, H. (1996). *La comunidad virtual: Una sociedad sin fronteras* [The virtual community: Homesteading on the electronic frontier]. Barcelona: Gedisa. (Original work published in 1993.)

Rodriquez, J. (2013). Narrating dementia: Self and community in an online forum. *Qualitative Health Research*, 23(9), 1215–1227.

Silverman, P.R. (1980). *Mutual help groups: Organization and development.* London: Sage.

Sixsmith, J., and Murray, C.D. (2001). Ethical issues in the documentary data analysis of Internet posts and archives. *Qualitative Health Research*, 11(3), 423–432.

Turkle, S. (1995). *Life on the screen: Identity in the age of Internet.* New York: Simon & Schuster.

Wilson, S.M., and Peterson, L.C. (2002). The anthropology of online communities. *Annual Review of Anthropology, 31*, 449–467.

Woolgar, S. (2002). *Virtual society? Technology, cyberole, reality.* Oxford: Oxford University Press.

List of Contributors

Roberta Raffaeta
University of Trento, Italy

Franz Graf
University of Vienna, Austria

Bernhard Hadolt
University of Vienna, Austria

Monika Gritsch
University of Vienna, Austria

Prachatip Kata
University of Amsterdam, the
    Netherlands

Bodil Ludvigsen
University of Copenhagen,
    Denmark

Ivo Quaranta
University of Bologna, Italy

Sylvie Fortin
La Biennale de Montréal, Canada

Josiane Le Gall
University of Montreal, Canada

Julia Thiesbonenkamp-Maag
Heidelberg University, Germany

Martine Verwey
Swiss Academy of Humanities and
    Social Sciences, Switzerland

Claudie Haxaire
University of Western Brittany,
    France

Sylvie Fainzang
National Institute of Health and
    Medical Research, USA

Lina Masana
Bradford Teaching Hospitals NHS
    Foundation Trust, UK

Acknowledgements

This volume would not exist without the work and support of many people whom we thank here. It is based on the manifold contributions of the participants of the 7th biannual conference of the Medical Anthropology At Home (MAAH) network held in 2012 in Driebergen, The Netherlands. The chapters themselves and the selection of the contributions more generally have greatly benefited from the intense engagement of the participants who read all presented papers ahead of the conference and advanced our discussions as discussants and through their critical questions and comments. We thank Rosalijn Both and Christopher Pell who were of tremendous help in organizing the conference. We also wish to acknowledge several individuals whose help has been essential for the further editorial process: Erin Martineau for her careful proofreading and copyediting, and Floortje Opbroek for making the index. Martine de Rooij and Hayley Murray have provided invaluable assistance in pulling together the volume and getting done the final manuscript preparation. Finally, we would also like to thank Jaap Wagenaar, our editor at Amsterdam University Press, for the extended support.

Bernhard Hadolt and Anita Hardon

Index